# Get the right

With the NHS these days, there are lots of choices. By making the right choice at the right time, you get the best possible treatment.

## Self-care

A well-stocked medicine cabinet will help you treat many everyday illnesses at home (see page 127 'Medicine chest').

## Pharmacy

Pharmacists (sometimes called Chemists) can offer advice on medicines and how to take them. They can also offer advice on common complaints, such as coughs, colds, aches and pains, and other health issues, such as healthy eating and giving up smoking. You can talk to your pharmacist in confidence – even about the most personal symptoms. Most pharmacies now have a quiet area away from other customers where you can speak to the pharmacist more privately.

## NHS Direct

**NHS Direct** is a 24-hour advice and health information service, staffed by nurses and professional advisors, providing confidential information on: ■ what to do if you or a family member feels ill; ■ particular health conditions; ■ local health services (such as doctors, dentists or out of hours pharmacies); and ■ self-help or support organisations. You can call **NHS Direct** on **0845 4647**. Calls are charged at local rates. For patients' safety, all calls are recorded.

## Your GP surgery

Your local GP surgery provides a range of services, including: ■ general medical advice and treatment; ■ prescriptions; ■ referral to a specialist or a hospital; ■ immunisations; and ■ tests. Out of normal surgery hours, all GPs have an emergency service. This service is only for urgent medical problems that cannot wait to be treated until normal surgery hours. However, if you are still not sure about the best way to deal with your symptoms, **NHS Direct** can advise you on what to do.

## NHS Walk-in Centres

NHS Walk-in Centres offer fast and convenient access to healthcare advice and treatments for minor injuries and illnesses. NHS Walk-in Centres do not replace local GP or hospital services but support existing local services. They are open from 7am until 10pm, seven days a week, and you do not need an appointment. Assessments are carried out by experienced NHS nurses who provide a skilled, safe and caring environment. To find out if there is a NHS Walk-in Centre near you, call **NHS Direct** on **0845 4647**.

## Accident and Emergency (999)

When it comes to your health or the health of someone in your family, it is often very obvious if the person is seriously ill and needs emergency care. You should get medical attention by either taking the patient to accident and emergency (A and E) or phoning 999 for an emergency ambulance (see page 128 'What is an emergency?').

# How to use this guide

This guide covers the most common symptoms which people call **NHS Direct** about for advice. It does not claim to cover all health problems but it is a handy reference for the most common symptoms that could affect you or your family. If this guide does not cover your particular symptom, call **NHS Direct** for advice.

■ Use the **Body key** (page 3) to help you find what symptoms you might have. The **Index** (pages 130 to 136) may also help you.

■ Turn to the section of the guide which covers those symptoms.

■ Answer the series of questions about your symptoms and follow the advice given.

■ If the guide directs you somewhere else within the guide, turn to that page and work through the questions in the same way.

■ The **Glossary of conditions** (pages 92 to 115) will give you general advice about particular conditions.

Your answers will give you three courses of action.

➕ **Self-care** – it's safe to manage this problem yourself.

🔧 **Call NHS Direct** – the **NHS Direct** nurse will be able to advise you on whether you need medical attention and, if you do, how quickly you should get help.

999 **Dial 999** – you need emergency help now.

If the guide suggests dealing with the problem yourself, it will give you advice on:

■ what to do;

■ what medicines, if any, you can buy from your pharmacist or chemist which could help; and

■ other people or organisations who may be able to offer more advice.

It is not always that easy to decide whether you have an emergency on your hands or not, which is why you may find calling **NHS Direct** helpful. For more advice see 'What is an emergency?' (pages 128 and 129).

## NHS Direct Online

You can also find the **NHS Direct self-help guide** on the Internet at **www.nhsdirect.nhs.uk**. **NHS Direct Online** also includes:
■ information on conditions and treatments;
■ advice on healthy living;
■ an A-Z guide to NHS services; and
■ advice on health stories in the news.

Use this **body key** to find your starting point.
What part of the body has the problem?
The colour will then direct you to the section of the
guide where you will find advice.

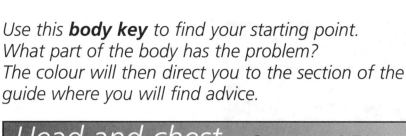

## Head and chest    *See pages 6-51*

Breast changes   *6-7*
Breathing difficulty in adults   *8-9*
Breathing difficulty in children   *10-11*
Chest pain in adults   *12-13*
Colds and flu   *14*
Coughing adults   *16-17*
Coughing children   *18-19*
Crying baby   *20-21*
Dizziness in adults   *22-23*
Earache in adults   *24-25*
Earache in children   *26-27*
Fever in adults   *28-29*
Fever in children   *30-31*
Hayfever   *15*

Headache in adults   *32-33*
Headache in children   *34-35*
Head injury in children   *36-37*
Poisoning   *38-39*
Sore mouth   *40-41*
Sore throat in adults   *42-43*
Toothache   *44-45*
Vomiting in adults   *46-47*
Vomiting in babies   *48-49*
Vomiting in children   *50-51*

## Abdomen    *See pages 52-77*

Absent periods   *52-53*
Adult vaginal bleeding   *54-55*
Backache in adults   *56-57*
Chest pain in adults   *12-13*
Diarrhoea in adults   *58-59*
Diarrhoea in babies and children   *60-61*
Erectile problems and impotence   *62-63*
Female abdominal pain in adults   *64-67*
Female urinary and vaginal problems in adults   *68-69*
Long-standing abdominal pain in adults   *70-71*
Male abdominal pain in adults   *72-73*
Male urinary and penile problems in adults   *74-75*
Poisoning   *38-39*
Tummy (abdominal) pain in children   *76-77*
Vomiting in adults   *46-47*
Vomiting in babies   *48-49*
Vomiting in children   *50-51*

## Limbs    *See pages 78-81*

Injuries to hands and feet   *78-79*
Joint pains   *80-81*

## Skin    *See pages 82-91*

Baby rashes   *82-83*
Burns and scalds   *84-85*
Itchy rashes   *86-87*
Rashes with fever   *88-89*
Rashes   *90-91*

# Is it a symptom or a condition?

*'I have another dose of the flu.'* How many times have you heard someone say this when they are actually suffering from a cold or are just feeling run-down? The names of some conditions tend to be used to describe how we feel rather than what we are suffering from.

**Symptom:**  A symptom is the personal effect a condition has on us. Feeling sick – nausea – is one of the symptoms of food poisoning, but it can also be a result of dehydration, travelling, ear infections, headaches – the list is almost endless.

**Condition:**  A condition is a collection of symptoms and describes what we are suffering from, such as flu, gastroenteritis and so on.

Pain is another good example of a symptom. No-one else can know how much pain you are suffering, and the way you suffer from pain is quite different from how other people experience it. Obviously pain can arise from a large number of conditions and injuries. 'Colic' is the description of one type of pain in the abdomen. It is not a condition itself and is the result of things like bowel irritation. Treating symptoms rather than the root cause of the problem – the condition – is common practice, not least because the condition is often long-standing or the precise cause of the symptom is not known. The truth of the matter is that, while we may not be able to cure all the conditions that affect us, we can provide treatments to make life more comfortable and pleasant. Rheumatoid arthritis is an example of this. Knowing the reason why we are suffering from certain symptoms, and telling the difference between a serious and a minor condition that is causing them, is important, and this guide will help you. If you are still not sure after using it, ring **NHS Direct** for advice.

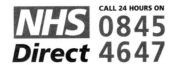

CALL 24 HOURS ON
0845 4647

www.nhsdirect.nhs.uk

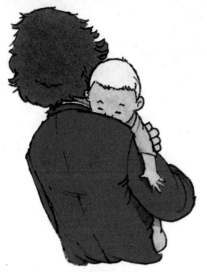

# How do I know if my baby is ill?

Parents are usually good at noticing when something is wrong with their baby. But it may be difficult to know what is wrong.

Here are some signs that can be important.

## 1. If your baby is not responding to you normally

– When awake, your baby may seem unusually drowsy or not interested in looking at you.

– Your baby may not be interested in feeding.

– Perhaps when cuddled, your baby feels floppy or limp.

– Your baby's cry seems different (perhaps moaning, whimpering or shrill), and soothing doesn't help.

If you think you notice these in your baby, please call **NHS Direct** and talk to a nurse.

## 2. Other signs of illness

If you are already worried and then notice other problems too (like those in the list below), call **NHS Direct** for advice.

– If your baby looks very pale.

– If your baby seems irritable and does not like being touched.

– If a new rash starts to appear.

– If your baby's skin looks bruised or discoloured.

– If your baby seems hot (feverish or has a temperature).

– If your baby seems breathless or is breathing much faster than usual.

– If your baby starts being sick (vomiting).

Remember, you know your baby better than anyone else!
If you are worried, call **NHS Direct** for advice.

## When taking a young child to hospital

If you and your child need to go to hospital:

– reassure your child and explain that you're going together to see the doctor at the hospital to make things better;

– take a favourite toy with you;

– dress your child in a coat or a dressing gown over their nightclothes, or dress your child fully (it doesn't matter which – do what seems most sensible);

– arrange care for other children or, if this is not possible, take them as well (it is not wise to leave a child at home without an adult there to look after them); and

– don't forget to leave a note, and take your keys, handbag or wallet with you.

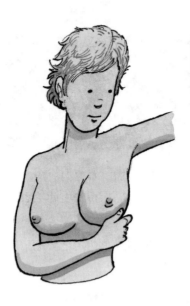

## Breast changes

Can you feel or see lumps, thickening, dimpling, puckering or depressions in the skin or changes in the general shape of the breast?

 **Yes**

**Call NHS Direct**

Most changes that take place in the breast are due to hormonal changes or ageing. Even so, these changes should be checked by a doctor or nurse.

See *Breast cancer* on page 92 for more information.

**No**

Do you experience pain or constant tenderness in your breast with each period?

 **Yes**

**Call NHS Direct**

Hormonal changes can produce tenderness for some women. If this has been happening for years, it is unlikely to be serious so wait until your period has finished and see if the tenderness or lumpiness is still there. If it is or if there is a sudden onset of pain with your periods, it should be checked by a doctor or nurse.

See *Breast cancer* on page 92 for more information.

**No**

Do you normally have lumps in your breasts that have been checked and found to be safe, but now find that a new lump has appeared?

 **Yes**

**Call NHS Direct**

Some women are prone to lumps in their breasts, but these can lead to a false sense of security. Each new lump should be examined by a doctor or nurse.

See *Breast cancer* on page 92 for more information.

**No**

*See the opposite page*

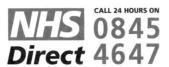
**NHS Direct** CALL 24 HOURS ON **0845 4647**

Is there any fluid when you squeeze the nipple or are you experiencing a discharge that is not breast milk?

 **Yes**

## Call NHS Direct

Some breast infections may cause these symptoms, but cancer can also do the same thing. It must be checked by a doctor or nurse.

See *Breast cancer* on page 92 for more information.

**No**

---

Do you have a strong family history of breast cancer – for example, has your mother or sister suffered from it?

 **Yes**

## Call NHS Direct

There is an increased risk of breast cancer if members of your family have suffered from it. You should discuss this with your doctor, who may recommend more regular medical examinations.

See *Breast cancer* on page 92 for more information.

**No**

---

Are you pregnant or have you just given birth?

 **Yes**

## Call NHS Direct

Major changes take place inside the breast during pregnancy, and will take place for quite a while even if you are not breast-feeding.

 **No**

---

### Self-care advice

- Often, tenderness and lumps in the breasts are related to your menstrual cycle (periods).
- Learn to examine your own breasts to find out what is normal for you.
- Keep a diary for a couple of months to see if the problem happens at the same time each month.
- If tenderness is causing discomfort, a simple painkiller, such as paracetamol, may help.
- Make sure the bra you are wearing fits properly.
- If the condition gets worse or new symptoms develop, call **NHS Direct**.
- If you are still worried or need further help, call **NHS Direct**.

**Before ringing NHS Direct or 999, it would be helpful if you think about the following and are ready to answer the questions if asked.**
- Your age or the age of the person you are calling about.
- Whether you or they are pregnant or have just given birth.
- Any medicines you or they are taking at the moment.
- Any serious illness you or they have had before.
- Whether any members of your or their family have suffered from breast cancer.

*Breast changes*

www.nhsdirect.nhs.uk

7

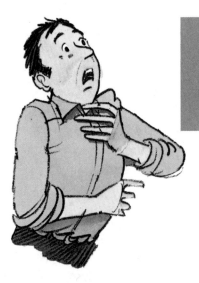

# Breathing difficulty in adults

Is there also a crushing chest pain which moves up to your jaw or left arm, makes you feel sick, has lasted more than 15 minutes or is not relieved by indigestion remedies?

 **Yes** → **Dial 999**

 **No**

Are your lips tinged blue, are you having difficulty speaking or are you wheezing?

 **Yes** → **Dial 999**

 **No**

Did the difficulty start after eating food, taking medicines or being bitten or stung by an insect?

 **Yes** → **Dial 999**

 **No**

Is there pain which is worse when you breathe in?

 **Yes** → **Call NHS Direct**

 **No**

*See the opposite page*

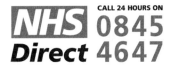 **CALL 24 HOURS ON** **NHS Direct** **0845 4647**

Did the breathing difficulty happen after some food, like bread, went 'down the wrong way'?

**Yes**  → **Dial 999**

 **No**

Is the breathing difficulty worse when you lie down?

**Yes**  → **Call NHS Direct**

 **No**

Is there also a fever, are you feeling flushed, hot and sweaty (is your temperature over 38°C or 100.4°F), is your phlegm green or does it contain blood?

**Yes**  → **Call NHS Direct**

 **No**

Has the difficulty gradually got worse over the past weeks?

**Yes**  → **Call NHS Direct**

 **No**

## Self-care advice

- If you are an asthmatic, take your inhalers (bronchodilators) as prescribed and call **NHS Direct** who will help to decide how urgent your condition is.
- If the condition gets worse or new symptoms develop, call **NHS Direct**.
- If you are still worried, call **NHS Direct**.

Before ringing **NHS Direct** or 999, it would be helpful if you think about the following and are ready to answer the questions if asked.
- How long you or the person you are calling about have been unwell.
- If it might be a heart attack.
- If you or they are very short of breath.
- Your temperature or their temperature (if possible).
- Any medicines you or they are taking at the moment.
- Any allergies you know of.
- Any illnesses, such as asthma or heart disease, you or they have had before.

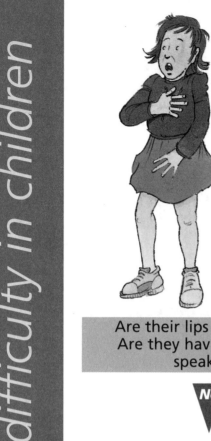

# Breathing difficulty in children

| | |
|---|---|
| Are their lips tinged blue? Are they having difficulty speaking? |  **Dial 999**  |

| | |
|---|---|
| Is the child wheezing? |  **Call NHS Direct**  |

| | |
|---|---|
| Did the breathing difficulty happen after some food, like bread, went 'down the wrong way'? |  **Dial 999**  |

| | |
|---|---|
| Did the difficulty start after taking medicine or being bitten or stung by an insect? |  **Dial 999**  |

*See the opposite page*

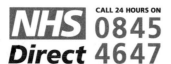

**NHS Direct** CALL 24 HOURS ON **0845 4647**

Is there also a fever, is the child flushed, or do they feel hot and sweaty (is the child's temperature over 38°C or 100.4°F)?

**Yes**

**Call NHS Direct**

**No**

### Self-care advice

- Breathing difficulties in children should not be ignored.
- If your child has asthma, make sure they take their inhalers (bronchodilators) as prescribed and call **NHS Direct** who will help to decide how urgent your child's condition is.
- If the condition gets worse or new symptoms develop, call **NHS Direct**.
- If you are still worried, call **NHS Direct**.

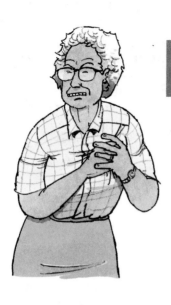

# Chest pain in adults

Have you felt this pain before during a heart attack?

 **Yes**

**Dial 999**

**Dial 999** now. Take any medicines they advise. It may only be angina but let the doctors decide.

 **No**

Do you have **any** of the following symptoms?
- Crushing pain like a tight band around your chest.
- Pain which moves to your jaw or left arm.
- Feeling sick.
- Sweating heavily.
- Short of breath.

 **Yes**

**Dial 999**

 **No**

Is the pain worse when you breathe in, is there green phlegm or is there blood in the phlegm?

 **Yes**

**Call NHS Direct**

 **No**

Do you have any difficulty in breathing?

 **Yes**

**Call NHS Direct**

 **No**

*See the opposite page*

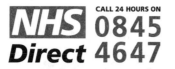
**NHS** CALL 24 HOURS ON **0845**
**Direct** **4647**

12

Do indigestion remedies (antacids) ease the pain?

 **Yes**

### Self-care

It may be indigestion. Take any indigestion remedies or **ask your pharmacist**, who will give good advice. If the pain fails to settle within 15 minutes, call **NHS Direct**.

 **No**

---

Is the pain worse when you bend over and is it eased by indigestion remedies (antacids)?

 **Yes**

### Call NHS Direct

Go to *Hiatus hernia* on page 98 for more information.

 **No**

---

Is the pain worse when you move your arms, or have you had unusual or strenuous exercise recently?

 **Yes**

### Self-care

You probably have muscle strain. **Ask your pharmacist** for advice.

 **No**

---

### Call NHS Direct

If you cannot sort out what to do from this list, please call **NHS Direct**.

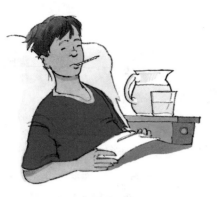

# Colds and flu

*This advice is suitable for children and adults.*

Are you developing a rash that does not fade when you press a glass tumbler or finger against it?

**Yes**  **Dial 999**

**No**

Is there sneezing, a runny nose, a mild temperature, a sore throat, and general aches and pains?

**Yes**

## Self-care

It could be a common cold which antibiotics cannot treat effectively. Unless the person is very old, frail or has some other serious condition, you **do not need to see your doctor**. Take paracetamol (or, for children, Calpol), warm soothing drinks and rest. **Ask your pharmacist** for advice.

**No**

Are you feeling flushed, hot and sweaty? Do you have a high temperature (over 38°C or 100.4°F), a headache, as well as a runny nose and general aches and pains?

**Yes**

## Self-care

It could be flu, which is generally worse than the common cold but is not helped with antibiotics. Paracetamol (or, for children, Calpol), warm drinks, and plenty of rest all help. Only groups such as young children, babies and elderly or frail people who have symptoms which are severe or do not go away need to call **NHS Direct**. However, if you are breathless, if it is painful to bend your neck or if light hurts your eyes, call **NHS Direct**.

**No**

## Self-care advice

- Take simple painkillers such as paracetamol (or, for children, Calpol) – this will help to bring your or their temperature down.
- Increase how much fluid you or they drink.
- Some people find that a simple cough medicine helps to soothe a ticklish dry cough.
- Flu vaccination for people who are at risk is important. People most at risk include the elderly, people with chronic illnesses such as heart, kidney or lung disease, people with reduced immunity (for example, people with HIV or having chemotherapy), and people living in nursing, residential or long-stay homes.
- If the condition gets worse or other symptoms develop, call **NHS Direct**.

**NHS** CALL 24 HOURS ON
**Direct** 0845 4647

# Hay fever

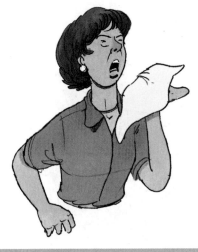

*The advice is suitable for children and adults.*

---

**Are you very short of breath?**  **Yes**

### Call NHS Direct

You should call **NHS Direct** as you may have asthma.

See ***Breathing difficulties*** on pages 8 to 11 for more information.

 **No**

---

**Do the symptoms (runny nose, sneezing, watery eyes) come on at a particular time of year?**  **Yes**

### Self-care

It is probably hay fever. Watch out for the pollen count, which is published in many newspapers. There are medicines that will help, particularly if taken early. **Ask your pharmacist** for advice.

 **No**

---

**Do the symptoms come on when you are in a particular place such as in a garden, in a workplace or near animals?**  **Yes**

### Self-care

It is probably an allergy to specific things such as bird droppings, dust or plants. Your pharmacist can advise you.

 **No**

---

**Do you develop the symptoms when you come home?**  **Yes**

### Self-care

You may be allergic to house mites. Try using a filter on the vacuum cleaner.

 **No**

---

### Call NHS Direct

If you are not sure what to do from this list, please call **NHS Direct**.

---

**Before ringing NHS Direct or 999, it would be helpful if you think about the following and are ready to answer the questions if asked.**

- How long you or the person you are calling about have been unwell.
- If you or they are very short of breath.
- Any medicines you or they are taking at the moment.
- Any allergies you know of.
- Any illnesses, such as asthma, you or they have had before.

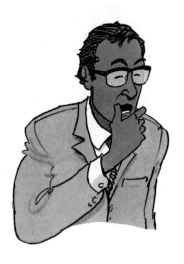

# Coughing adults

Are you severely short of breath, do you have a blue tinge to your lips or a severe pain in your chest?

**Yes**  **Dial 999**

**No**

Did you have a coughing fit after some food, like bread or peanuts, went 'down the wrong way'?

**Yes**  **Dial 999**

**No**

Have you recently breathed in any toxic fumes, such as petrol, ammonia or industrial chemicals?

**Yes**  **Call NHS Direct**

These chemicals can badly irritate the lungs.

**No**

Did the cough come on after taking some new medicine?

**Yes**  **Call NHS Direct**

Some medicines can cause a cough and even breathing difficulties. Call **NHS Direct**.

**No**

Is there severe pain when you cough?

**Yes**  **Call NHS Direct**

**No**

Is there a wheeze?

**Yes**  **Call NHS Direct**

It may be an asthmatic attack. If there is any shortness of breath, you should call **NHS Direct**.

**No**

*See the opposite page*

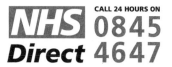

CALL 24 HOURS ON
**0845 4647**

Is there any blood
in your phlegm?

**Yes**

**Call NHS Direct**

**No**

Is the phlegm green?

**Yes**

**Call NHS Direct**

You may have a chest infection.
Call **NHS Direct**.

**No**

Has the cough lasted for many
weeks or are you losing weight?

**Yes**

**Call NHS Direct**

Some chest infections can last for
a long time. Call **NHS Direct**.

**No**

Is there a fever, are you feeling
flushed, hot and sweaty (is your
temperature over 38°C or 100.4°F),
do you have a runny nose,
sneezing, a sore throat or general
aches and pains?

**Yes**

**Self-care**

You probably have a cold which will not be
helped by antibiotics. Paracetamol will reduce
the fever. Use warm honey and lemon drinks to
soothe the cough. Cough medicines may be of
some value. **Ask your pharmacist** for advice.

Go to *Colds and flu* on
page 14 for more
information.

**No**

Do you or does anyone around
you smoke?

**Yes**

**Self-care**

Smoking or passive smoking can affect
you even if it is not taking place in the
same room as you.

See *Smoking and
lung cancer* on page 112
for more information.

**No**

### Self-care advice

- Drink lots of fluids.
- Avoid a smoky atmosphere.
- A home remedy of one teaspoon of
  honey in a small glass of warm water
  sometimes helps.
- Stay in a warm, humid environment
  such as a bathroom with the shower
  on.
- If the condition gets worse or new
  symptoms develop, call **NHS Direct**.
- If you are still worried, call
  **NHS Direct**.

**Before ringing NHS Direct or 999, it
would be helpful if you think about
the following and are ready to answer
the questions if asked.**

- How long you or the person you are
  calling about have been unwell.
- Your temperature or their
  temperature (if possible).
- If you or they are very short of breath.
- If there is anyone else in the house
  with the same problem.
- If there is bloodied or green phlegm.
- When you or they last had anything
  to eat or drink.
- Any medicines you or they are
  taking at the moment.
- Any allergies you know of.
- Any illness, such as asthma or
  bronchitis, you or they have had before.

Coughing adults

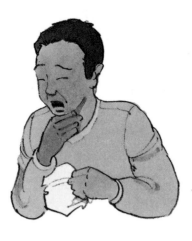

# Coughing children

*Before going through
the following questions, check
'How do I know if my baby is ill?'
on page 5.*

Are they having difficulty breathing or are their lips blue?  **Yes**

**Dial 999**

For whatever reason the child is not getting enough air. **Dial 999**

 **No**

Did they have a coughing fit after some food, like bread or peanuts, went 'down the wrong way'?  **Yes**

**Dial 999**

An obstruction of the airway may cause this kind of coughing. **Dial 999**

 **No**

Does your child vomit after a coughing fit with a whooping noise?  **Yes**

**Call NHS Direct**

It could be whooping cough (pertussis). Give paracetamol (for example, Calpol) and put a bowl of water in the room to humidify the air. Call **NHS Direct**.

 **No**

Is there any blood in their phlegm?  **Yes**

**Call NHS Direct**

Repeated coughing can cause small blood vessels to burst. Call **NHS Direct**.

 **No**

*See the opposite page*

**NHS** CALL 24 HOURS ON
**Direct** **0845 4647**

Does your child have **any** of the following symptoms?
- A runny nose.
- A sore throat.
- A fever. Is the child flushed, do they feel hot and sweaty (is the child's temperature over 38°C or 100.4°F)?
- General aches and pains.
- Are they sneezing?

 **Yes**

### Self-care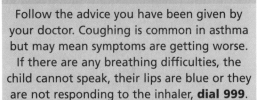

It is probably a cold or flu.
**Ask your pharmacist** for advice.

 **No**

Does your child have asthma?

**Yes**

### Self-care

Follow the advice you have been given by your doctor. Coughing is common in asthma but may mean symptoms are getting worse. If there are any breathing difficulties, the child cannot speak, their lips are blue or they are not responding to the inhaler, **dial 999**.

 **No**

Is the cough worse when people smoke?

**Yes**

### Self-care

Passive smoking affects children even if they are not in the same room as you, especially if they already have some other condition like a cold or asthma.
*Either smoke outside or give it up.*

Go to *Smoking and lung cancer* on page 112 for more information.

 **No**

### Self-care advice

- Give the child extra fluids.
- Avoid a smoky atmosphere.
- Some people find the home remedy of one teaspoon of honey in a small glass of warm water sometimes helps.
- Babies often cope better if they sit up.
- Stay with the child in a warm, humid environment such as a bathroom with the shower on.
- If the condition gets worse or new symptoms develop, call **NHS Direct**.
- If you are still worried, call **NHS Direct**.

Before ringing **NHS Direct** or 999, it would be helpful if you think about the following and are ready to answer the questions if asked.
- How long they have been unwell.
- If they are very short of breath.
- Their temperature (if possible).
- If there is anyone else in the house with the same problem.
- When they last had anything to eat or drink.
- Any medicines they are taking at the moment.
- Any allergies you know of.
- Any illnesses, such as asthma, they have had before.

www.nhsdirect.nhs.uk

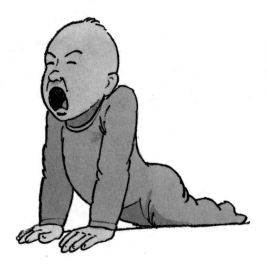

# Crying baby

*Before going through
the following questions, check
'How do I know if my baby is ill?'
on page 5.*

| | | |
|---|---|---|
| Does your baby have a rash? |  **Yes** | **Call NHS Direct**  |

 **No**

| | | |
|---|---|---|
| Do they have a fever, is the child flushed, do they feel hot and sweaty (is the child's temperature over 38°C or 100.4°F)? |  **Yes** | **Call NHS Direct**  |

 **No**

| | | |
|---|---|---|
| Does your baby cry while feeding on a bottle? |  **Yes** | **Self-care** ✚ |

 **No**

*See the opposite page*

**Self-care**

The teat hole may be too small. Try a larger teat hole. Or, the baby may have a blocked nose and not be able to breathe properly while feeding. **Ask your health visitor** for advice.

**NHS Direct** CALL 24 HOURS ON **0845 4647**

Are you able to find a way of soothing your baby?

 **Yes**

 **No**

## Self-care advice

- If you think the child may be hungry, try to give them some of their normal food.
- You may be able to soothe the child by taking them for a ride in their buggy or in a car.
- If the baby's crying does not settle or the baby seems ill, call **NHS Direct**.
- If you are still worried, call **NHS Direct**.

## Self-care

Your baby may have colic. No-one knows the cause of colic. It is not due to bad parenting but parents often feel they must be doing something wrong. Gentle soothing and rocking may help your baby relax and settle down. Once your baby has stopped crying and is drowsy, put them down to sleep. If your baby starts crying again, leave them for 10 to 15 minutes before trying to soothe them again. Although crying can be reduced, it is much easier to cope with if it can be shared. Even if you can't get someone to help you at home, try to talk about your feelings. **Your doctor, practice nurse or health visitor** will understand how hard it can be to deal with a crying baby who is otherwise healthy and well.

*Crying baby*

www.nhsdirect.nhs.uk

21

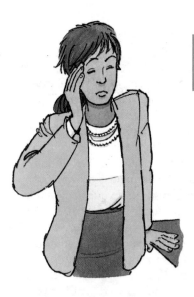

# Dizziness in adults

Is there any weakness, numbness or tingling in any of your limbs, are strange things happening with your sight, or do you have a severe headache or are you having difficulty speaking properly?

 **Yes**

### Call NHS Direct

There are a number of things which will cause dizziness and if you feel dizzy along with these other symptoms, it needs to be checked by a doctor or nurse.
Call **NHS Direct**.

 **No**

Did the dizziness follow a recent blow to the head and it has not gone away?

 **Yes**

### Call NHS Direct

Some blows to the head can cause a build-up of pressure in the skull. Call **NHS Direct**.

 **No**

Is the dizziness made worse by holding your head in a certain way or moving your head to a certain position?

 **Yes**

### Call NHS Direct

Some problems with the ear's balancing mechanism can cause this. Call **NHS Direct**.

 **No**

*See the opposite page*

**NHS Direct**
CALL 24 HOURS ON
**0845 4647**

Is there pain in the ear, a loss of hearing or a strange noise which won't go away?

 **Yes**

## Call NHS Direct

Some ear infections will cause these effects. Call **NHS Direct**.

 **No**

## Self-care advice ✚

■ Take things very carefully – try not to make sudden movements.
■ The person with dizziness should not drive a vehicle.
■ If the condition gets worse or new symptoms develop, call **NHS Direct**.
■ If you are still worried, call **NHS Direct**.

**Before ringing NHS Direct or 999, it would be helpful if you think about the following and are ready to answer the questions if asked.**

■ How long you or the person you are calling about have been unwell and whether it followed a recent head injury.
■ If there is any weakness or change of feeling in any limbs.
■ Your temperature or their temperature (if possible).
■ If there is any neck pain.
■ If there is any pain in the ear.
■ If you or they are confused, drowsy or vomiting.
■ If there is anyone else in the house with the same problem.
■ When you or they last had anything to eat or drink.
■ Any medicines you or they are taking at the moment.
■ Any illnesses, such as ear infections, which you or they have had before.

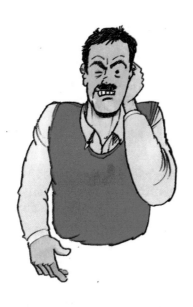

# Earache in adults

Is the pain very severe or is there vomiting or a yellow discharge from your ear?

 **Yes**

### Call NHS Direct
You may have an infection of the middle ear. Call **NHS Direct**.

 **No**

Is there also pain in your teeth or jaw?

 **Yes**

### Call NHS Direct
You may have a dental abscess or a bad tooth. Call **NHS Direct**.

 **No**

Is there itchiness just inside your ear or is the pain worse when your pull your ear lobe?

 **Yes**

### Call NHS Direct
You may have an infection of the outer part of the ear. Call **NHS Direct**.

 **No**

Is your hearing dull, does it change as you move your head or did the pain come on after a bath or swimming?

 **Yes**

### Self-care
There may be wax against your eardrum, with water held inside the ear that causes hearing dullness and pain. **Ask your pharmacist** for advice.

 **No**

Do you have a cold or hay fever?

 **Yes**

### Self-care
The tube which connects the back of the ear to the throat keeps the pressure the same on both sides. It gets blocked during a cold. Try swallowing hard while holding your nose. Your pharmacist will advise you on decongestants to use.

 **No**

*See the opposite page*

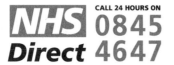

**NHS** CALL 24 HOURS ON **0845**
**Direct** **4647**

**Did the pain start during or after a plane trip?**  **Yes**

**No**

### Self-care

There may have been unequal pressure on each side of the eardrum. This happens more often when you have a cold or an ear infection. Try swallowing hard while holding your nose. Take paracetamol. If the pain does not go away after two days, **speak to your doctor**.

**Did the pain start after trying to clean out wax with your finger or some other object?**  **Yes**

**No**

### Call NHS Direct

You may have damaged the sensitive lining of the ear or even the eardrum itself. The smallest thing you should put in your ear is your elbow! Never use cotton buds to clear out wax as they only push the wax further in and may cause damage to the inside of your ear.

### Self-care advice +

- Try simple painkillers.
- If the cold or wind makes your earache worse, cover your ears with a hat or a scarf.
- If the condition gets worse or new symptoms develop, call **NHS Direct**.
- If you are still worried, call **NHS Direct**.

*Earache in adults*

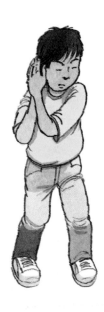

# Earache in children

Has your child injured their ear or stuck something into it? — **Yes**  → **Call NHS Direct**

 **No**

Is your child very distressed, with pain that has not been helped by painkillers such as paracetamol (for example, Calpol)? — **Yes**  → **Call NHS Direct**

 **No**

Is there yellow or blood-stained liquid (a discharge) coming from the ear? — **Yes**  → **Call NHS Direct**

 **No**

Do you think your child is getting worse? — **Yes**  → **Call NHS Direct**

 **No**

*See the opposite page*

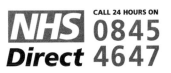
**NHS Direct** CALL 24 HOURS ON **0845 4647**

| Has your child got lumps behind their ear? | **Yes** ▶ | **Call NHS Direct**  |
| --- | --- | --- |

**No** ▼

## Self-care advice

Earache is a common and unpleasant symptom in childhood.

Most ear infections will clear up on their own but there are ways you can help relieve the symptoms.

- A painkiller, such as children's paracetamol (for example, Calpol), will help relieve the pain.
- Place your child in an upright position with pillows.
- A warm hot-water bottle wrapped in a towel placed over the infected ear may give some pain relief.
- Keep your child away from smoky environments.
- Don't let your child drink from a bottle while they are lying down.
- Don't give decongestants as they will not help to relieve symptoms.
- Never poke any objects into the ear (for example, cotton buds) as they often pack the wax tighter and can damage the ear.
- If the condition gets worse or new symptoms develop, call **NHS Direct**.
- If you are still worried, call **NHS Direct**.

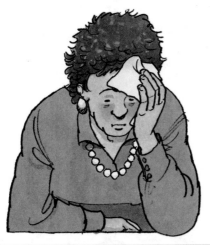

# Fever in adults

*You may have a fever if you are feeling flushed, hot and sweaty (if your temperature is over 38°C or 100.4°F).*

Is it painful to bend your neck or does light hurt your eyes?  **Yes**  **Call NHS Direct**

 **No**

Have you recently travelled abroad?  **Yes**  **Call NHS Direct**

 **No**

Do you have a severe headache or are you vomiting continuously?  **Yes**  **Call NHS Direct**

 **No**

Are you short of breath, is it painful to breathe in, or is there green phlegm?  **Yes**  **Call NHS Direct**

 **No**

Do you have a rash?  **Yes** Go to *Rashes with fever* on page 88 for more information.

 **No**

Is there a severe pain in your back?  **Yes**  **Call NHS Direct**

 **No**

*See the opposite page*

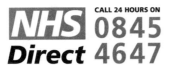 **CALL 24 HOURS ON** **0845 4647**

**Are you vomiting or do you have diarrhoea?**  **Yes** ▶

### Self-care ✚

You may have food poisoning or a stomach bug. If the vomiting and diarrhoea is mild, **ask your pharmacist** for advice. **If it is severe, call NHS Direct**.

**No** ▼

**Do you have general aches and pains, a sore throat, a runny nose or sneezing?**  **Yes** ▶

### Self-care ✚

You probably have a viral infection such as a cold or flu. **Ask your pharmacist** for advice.

 **No** ▼

### Self-care advice ✚

- Try resting in bed if possible.
- Wear light clothing only.
- Take paracetamol or ibuprofen (follow the manufacturer's instructions) to help keep the temperature down. If you are pregnant, do not take ibuprofen and only take paracetamol as instructed.
- Drink more fluids.
- Make sure the room temperature is not too warm.
- If the condition gets worse or new symptoms develop, call **NHS Direct**.
- If you are still worried, call **NHS Direct**.

**Before ringing NHS Direct or 999, it would be helpful if you think about the following and are ready to answer the questions if asked.**

- How long you or the person you are calling about have been unwell.
- If you or they have recently travelled abroad.
- If there is a red or purple rash, if light hurts the eyes or if there is pain when bending the neck.
- If you or they are very short of breath.
- Your temperature or their temperature (if possible).
- If there is anyone else in the house with the same problem.
- When you or they last had anything to eat or drink.
- Any medicines you or they are taking at the moment.

www.nhsdirect.nhs.uk

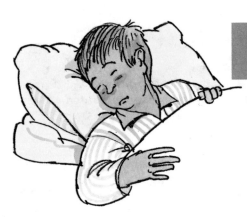

# Fever in children

*Your child may have a fever if they are flushed or feel hot and sweaty (if their temperature is over 38°C or 100.4°F).*

Is your child under one year old?  **Yes**  **Call NHS Direct**

 **No**

Do they have a rash?  **Yes** Go to *Rashes with fever* on page 88 for more information.

 **No**

Do they have difficulty breathing?  **Yes**  **Call NHS Direct**

 **No**

Is your child difficult to wake, not taking or keeping down fluids, or complaining of the light hurting their eyes?  **Yes** **Call NHS Direct**

The child may have an infection. Call **NHS Direct**.

 **No**

Do they also have diarrhoea?  **Yes** Go to *Diarrhoea in babies and children* on page 60 for more information.

**No**

*See the opposite page*

**NHS Direct**
CALL 24 HOURS ON
**0845 4647**

Are there any tender swellings around their jaw and neck?

**Yes**

### Self-care

It is probably swollen glands. Give the child paracetamol (for example, Calpol) and **ask your pharmacist** for advice. If the symptoms continue, **speak to your doctor**.

**No**

Do they have earache?

**Yes**

Go to *Earache in children* on page 26 for more information.

**No**

Do they have a sore throat, a cough or a runny nose, or are they sneezing?

**Yes**

### Self-care

It is probably a cold or flu. **Ask your pharmacist** for advice.

**No**

Is there pain in the tummy (abdomen)?

**Yes**

Go to *Tummy (abdominal) pain in children* on page 76 for more information.

**No**

Has the fever lasted more than five days?

**Yes**

### Call NHS Direct

**No**

### Self-care advice

- Regularly give your child paracetamol (for example, Calpol) to reduce the temperature (check the instructions on the packet for the right dose).
- Give them an extra amount of their favourite cool drink or ice lollies.
- Make sure your child is not overdressed – a vest and nappy or pants is enough clothing for them as long as the house is at the normal room temperature.
- Cover your child in a light cotton sheet when they are in bed.
- If the condition gets worse or new symptoms develop, call **NHS Direct**.
- Make sure your child is up to date with all their immunisations.
- If you are still worried, call **NHS Direct**.

**Before ringing NHS Direct or 999**, it would be helpful if you think about the following and are ready to answer the questions if asked.
- How long they have been unwell.
- If they are short of breath.
- Their temperature (if possible).
- If there is a red or purple rash, if light hurts their eyes, if they are drowsy or if bending their neck is painful.
- If there is anyone else in the house with the same problem.
- When they last had anything to eat or drink.
- Any medicines they are taking at the moment.

*Fever in children*

www.nhsdirect.nhs.uk

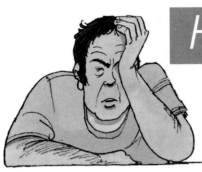

# Headache in adults

Are you developing a rash that does not fade when you press a glass tumbler or finger against it?

 **Yes** → **Dial 999**

 **No**

Do you have **any** of the following symptoms?
- A fever, feeling flushed, hot and sweaty (your temperature is over 38°C or 100.4°F).
- The light hurts your eyes.
- It hurts to bend your neck.

 **Yes** → There is more advice in *Fever in adults* but if the pain is severe, stop answering the questions and call **NHS Direct**.

Go to *Fever in adults* on page 28 for more information.

 **No**

Have you had a recent blow to your head and are you now becoming drowsy or confused or are you vomiting?

 **Yes** → **Dial 999**

Most serious head injuries will affect the person within 24 hours but some will take longer. **Dial 999**.

 **No**

Is the pain behind one eye or is your vision affected?

 **Yes** → **Call NHS Direct**

 **No**

Are there visual patterns?

 **Yes** → **Call NHS Direct**

You may have a migraine. There are treatments **from your pharmacist** which will help or reduce the severity of the symptoms. Call **NHS Direct**.

 **No**

*See the opposite page*

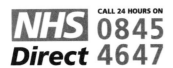

**NHS Direct** CALL 24 HOURS ON **0845 4647**

Did the headache start after you had drunk a lot of alcohol? **Yes**

**No**

## Self-care

Hangover headaches can be severe but usually respond to plenty of fluids and paracetamol. Your pharmacist will advise.

Go to *Hangovers* on page 97 for more information.

---

Is there any change in your vision, hearing, taste or balance, or are you vomiting more? **Yes**

**No**

## Call NHS Direct

---

Is your headache worse when you bend forward? **Yes**

**No**

## Self-care

You may have sinusitis – an infection of the spaces in the bones of the face. Take strong painkillers according to the manufacturer's instructions and ring **NHS Direct**.

---

Is the headache worse during stress or anxiety such as while at work or during stressful times at home? **Yes**

**No**

## Self-care

It could be a stress headache which will respond well to either avoiding, or dealing with, those things causing the stress, or better coping methods such as relaxation techniques. Ask your practice nurse about relaxation techniques. Paracetamol will help in the short term but you should not use it regularly.

---

## Self-care advice

- A common cause of early-morning headaches is grinding your teeth at night. You should **see your dentist**.
- Take regular painkillers, such as paracetamol, following the manufacturer's instructions for correct doses.
- Wrapping a warm towel around your neck may help relieve headaches caused by tension.
- Sometimes a cold flannel placed on the area of the pain can be soothing.
- If new symptoms develop, your headache gets worse or does not go away, call **NHS Direct**.
- Caffeine may sometimes cause headaches. Reduce the amount of coffee and tea you drink.
- If you are still worried, call **NHS Direct**.

**Before ringing NHS Direct or 999, it would be helpful if you think about the following and are ready to answer the questions if asked.**
- Your symptoms (the questions you answered 'Yes' to), or the symptoms of the person you are calling about.
- Your temperature or their temperature (if possible).
- When you or they last had anything to eat or drink.
- Any medicines you or they are taking at the moment.
- Any allergies you know of.
- Any serious illnesses you or they have had before.

*Headache in adults*

# *Headache in children*

Is your child developing a rash that does not fade when you press a glass tumbler or finger against it?

 **Yes** → **Dial 999**

 **No**

Does your child have **any** of the following symptoms?
- A fever, is flushed, and feels hot and sweaty (your child's temperature is over 38°C or 100.4°F).
- The light hurts your child's eyes.
- It hurts to bend their neck.

**Yes** → **Call NHS Direct**

Stop answering the questions and call **NHS Direct**.

 **No**

Has there been a recent blow to the head and your child is now becoming drowsy or confused or is vomiting?

**Yes** → **Call NHS Direct**

Most serious head injuries will affect the child within 24 hours but some will take longer. Call **NHS Direct**.

 **No**

Is there also pain or discharge from inside one ear?

 **Yes** →

They may have an ear infection.

Go to *Earache in children* on page 26 for more information.

 **No**

Is your child having problems with their vision?

 **Yes** → **Call NHS Direct**

They may have a migraine, which can run in families. There are treatments from your doctor which will prevent or reduce the severity of the symptoms. Call **NHS Direct**.

 **No**

*See the opposite page*

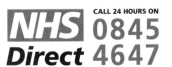 **CALL 24 HOURS ON 0845 4647**

34

Has the headache been getting worse or more frequent over the past weeks?

**Yes**  **Call NHS Direct**

 **No**

Does the headache only start before they are about to go to school or after they come home?

**Yes**

**Self-care**

It could be stress or anxiety about school or the pressure of homework. A chat with their teacher may help. In the short term, paracetamol (for example, Calpol) may ease the symptoms but you should not use it regularly.

 **No**

Is there also tooth or jaw pain?

**Yes**

**Self-care**

Bad teeth can cause headaches. **Ask your dentist** for advice.

 **No**

Has your child missed breakfast or any midday meals?

**Yes**

**Self-care**

It is important that your child eats regular meals as missing out on early meals can cause a headache. Give them some bread and milk. Avoid foods that contain a lot of sugar.

**No**

### Self-care advice

- Try giving your child paracetamol (for example, Calpol) according to the manufacturer's instructions. If, after taking paracetamol, the headache continues for 24 hours, call **NHS Direct**.
- If the condition gets worse or any other symptoms develop, call **NHS Direct**.
- If you are still worried, call **NHS Direct**.

Before ringing **NHS Direct** or 999, it would be helpful if you think about the following and are ready to answer the questions if asked.
- Their symptoms (the questions you answered 'Yes' to).
- Their temperature (if possible).
- When they last had anything to eat or drink.
- Any medicines they are taking at the moment.
- Any allergies you know of.
- Any serious illnesses they have had before.

## Headache in children

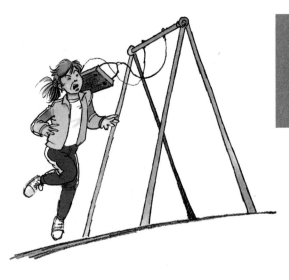

# Head injury in children

Is your child unconscious?  **Yes**  **Dial 999** 999

If the injury was only to the head,
lie them on one side, with a cushion
at their back, their upper knee brought
forward, and their head pointing downward
to allow any vomit to escape without them
swallowing it or breathing it in.
If there is any danger of a neck injury or
spine injury, do not move them. **Dial 999**.

 **No**

Did your child become
unconscious or did they seem
dazed or groggy immediately
after the injury?  **Yes**  **Dial 999** 999

Any loss of consciousness needs to be
checked. **Dial 999**.

 **No**

Did they have a fit, a turn or a
convulsion immediately after the
injury or at any time since?  **Yes**  **Dial 999** 999

Any fit should be checked by a doctor or
nurse. **Dial 999**.

 **No**

Are they deaf in one ear
or seeing double?  **Yes**  **Call NHS Direct**

 **No**

*See the opposite page*

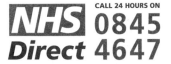 **NHS Direct** CALL 24 HOURS ON **0845 4647**

Have they vomited more than twice since the accident?  **Yes**

 **No**

### Call NHS Direct

Head injuries do tend to make children vomit but they should stop soon afterwards. If the vomiting starts later, or happens more than twice, call **NHS Direct**.

Are they increasingly dazed or groggy afterwards?  **Yes**

**No**

### Call NHS Direct

Children tend to sleep after a head injury. This is fine as long as you can wake them every hour for the first six hours after the injury or they are not vomiting. Otherwise call **NHS Direct**.

### Self-care advice ✚

- Place a cold facecloth over the bruised area.
- Give your child paracetamol (for example, Calpol) if you think they are in pain – read the instructions for the correct dose.
- Encourage your child to rest quietly for the next 48 hours and watch them for signs of getting worse. This may include frequent bouts of sickness and abnormal behaviour.
- If your child's symptoms worsen or any new symptoms develop, call **NHS Direct**.
- If you are still worried, call **NHS Direct**.

**Before ringing NHS Direct or 999, it would be helpful if you think about the following and are ready to answer the questions if asked.**

- If they are unconscious or were knocked out for a while.
- When the injury happened and how long they have been unwell.
- If there is a problem with their vision, hearing or balance.
- If they are vomiting, confused or very drowsy.
- If they had a fit afterwards.
- When they last had anything to eat or drink.
- Any medicines they are taking at the moment.

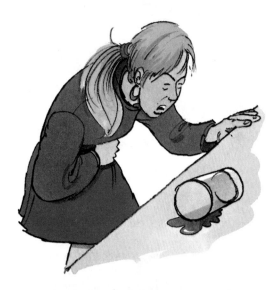

# Poisoning

*This advice is suitable for adults and children.*

Is the person very drowsy, unconscious or not able to breathe properly?

 **Yes**

### Dial 999

Lie them on their side, with a cushion behind their back and their upper leg pulled slightly forward so they don't fall on their face or roll backwards. Wipe any vomit away from their mouth. Keep their head pointing downward to allow any vomit to escape without them breathing it in or swallowing it. Don't give them anything to eat or drink. **Dial 999**.

 **No**

Is the substance they have swallowed in the following list?
Dishwashing products • Oven cleaner • Medicines • Drain cleaner • Ammonia • Rat or ant poisons • Mothballs • Weed-killer or pesticides • Windscreen washer fluid • Antifreeze

 **Yes**

### Dial 999

If they are very unwell, dial **999**. If they don't have any symptoms, call **NHS Direct**. Do not try to make them sick as it will make them worse.

 **No**

Is the substance they have swallowed in the following list?
**Household products:** Carpet cleaner • Fabric conditioner • Fabric washing powders or liquids • Hand washing-up liquid (not machine dishwasher products) • Liquid soap
**Cosmetics:** Baby oil • Baby wipes • Hair conditioner or shampoo (not medicated) • Moisturiser cream or lotion • Solid cosmetics (lipstick, make-up, eye shadow)
**DIY products:** Domestic *emulsion* paint • Putty • PVA (polyvinyl alcohol) glue • Wallpaper paste
**Garden:** Earth, soil or compost • Animal faeces (poo) are not 'poisonous' but may cause infections and if you are concerned, you should call **NHS Direct** • Worms, snails, tadpoles or slugs are not poisonous if eaten, although you may get bitten or stung by insects and spiders, which may be poisonous.

 **Yes**

### Self-care

These substances are not usually dangerous when they are taken accidentally.
Do not try to make the person sick as it will make them worse. Give them small sips of milk or water if they can swallow properly. Stay calm.
If they have swallowed a large amount or if you are worried about any symptoms they have, call **NHS Direct**.
Otherwise watch them carefully for the next four hours and care for them at home.

*Continued on the opposite page*

**NHS Direct** CALL 24 HOURS ON **0845 4647**

**Plants:** There are many plants that grow in the UK. Most are harmless or may cause only a mild stomach upset, for example, *Pyracantha*, *Cotoneaster* and honeysuckle (*Lonicera*). However, there are some types which can cause more serious trouble and it is important to identify the exact type of plant that may be causing concern, before you ring **NHS Direct**. You should try to know the types of plant growing in your own or shared garden. The scientific or Latin names are more useful and accurate if you can find them. • Fungi, mushrooms or toadstools are very difficult to identify and a few are very dangerous. If you are worried, then it is important to collect an example of the fungus that is involved and details about where it was found before you go to A and E. Never eat fungi as food unless you are absolutely sure that they are edible and have been reliably identified.

**Drugs and medicines:** Calamine lotion • Emollients (E45® preparations, petroleum jelly) • Evening primrose oil • Folic acid • Oral contraceptives and hormone replacement (HRT) preparations • Simple linctus • Steroid creams • Zinc oxide creams and lotions (for example, Sudocrem®)

**Miscellaneous:** Artificial sweeteners • Bird seed • Blu-Tack® and similar adhesives • Candles • Cat or dog food • Chalk • Coal • Crepe paper • Cut flower food • Expanded polystyrene • Felt tip or ballpoint pen ink • Fish food • House plant food (for example, Phostrogen®) • Ice-pack fluid (methylcellulose) • Matches • Nappies • Pencil 'leads' (graphite) • Plasticine® • Silica gel • Wax crayons

**No**

## Call NHS Direct

If you cannot sort out what to do from this list, please call **NHS Direct**.

**Before ringing NHS Direct or 999, it would be helpful if you think about the following and are ready to answer the questions if asked.**
- What the poison was.
- When they took the poison and, if possible, how much.
- If they are conscious.
- If they are very short of breath.
- Any medicines they are taking at the moment.
- Remember to take the container of poison and any medicines they are taking with you to hospital.

## Self-care advice

- Lock all chemicals and medicines out of sight of children.
- Keep all products in their original containers. Never put any medicines or chemicals, such as weedkiller, in soft-drink bottles.
- Never call medicines sweets.
- Clean out old medicines frequently and return them to your local pharmacist for them to get rid of safely.
- Rinse empty containers and throw them out in a safe place.
- Never take or give any medicines in the dark.
- Wherever possible buy products that have child-resistant caps.
- Store cleaning products out of reach and, where possible, out of sight of children.
- Don't store medicines or cleaning products near food.
- Keep the number of your family doctor and your local hospital ready to hand.
- Try taking a safety tour of your home with any young children and see if you can get them to point out the poisons.
- Ask the Royal Society for the Prevention of Accidents for advice on 0121 248 2000.

Below is a list of products that could be dangerous.
- Dishwashing products
- Oven cleaner
- Medicines
- Drain cleaner
- Ammonia
- Rat and ant poisons
- Mothballs
- Weedkiller and pesticides
- Windscreen washer fluid
- Antifreeze

www.nhsdirect.nhs.uk

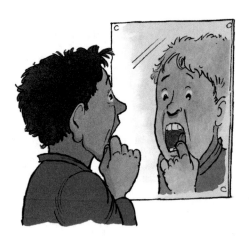

# Sore mouth

**Are there spots or discoloured patches inside your mouth?**

 Yes

## Call NHS Direct

If they are creamy yellow and scrape off leaving a raw area, it may be a thrush infection. If they do not scrape off, they are probably mouth ulcers. If the spots do not clear up after a couple of weeks, **speak to your doctor**.

See *Oral thrush* on page 114 and *Mouth ulcers* on page 107 for more information.

No

**Are your gums red, swollen and painful?**

 Yes

## Call NHS Direct

You may have a gum infection. You may have bad breath as well. **See your dentist.**

 No

**Is the pain and the spots or rash only at your lips?**

 Yes

## Call NHS Direct

If the rash is where your lip meets your skin, it is possibly a cold sore (herpes).

See *Cold sores* on page 93 for more information.

 No

**Are there painful cracks at the corners of your mouth?**

 Yes

## Call NHS Direct

In adults this can be caused by badly-fitting dentures or, more rarely, a vitamin deficiency. In children it is often caused by constantly licking at the edges of their mouth.

 No

*See the opposite page*

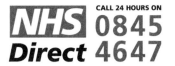

**NHS Direct** CALL 24 HOURS ON 0845 4647

Is the pain worse when you bite down, or is it only in one tooth? **Yes**

It may be an abscess or a bad tooth.
***Make an appointment with your dentist.***

Go to ***Toothache*** on page 44 for more information.

**No**

### Self-care advice ✚

- Drink plenty of fluids but make sure the drinks are not too hot or too cold as this could make the soreness feel worse.
- Avoid foods that may cause discomfort, such as highly-spiced foods or those containing salt or vinegar.
- Stick to soft foods to avoid scratching the inside of your mouth.
- Watch children to make sure that they do not put things in their mouth that could make the condition worse.
- Lozenges may help. Your pharmacist will be able to advise which would be the most suitable for you.
- Oral hygiene is very important. Make sure you brush your teeth at least twice a day and visit your dentist for a checkup every six months.
- If you are still suffering from a sore mouth after two weeks, or if the condition gets worse or new symptoms develop, **speak to your doctor** or call **NHS Direct**.
- If you are still worried or need further help, call **NHS Direct**.

**Before ringing NHS Direct or 999, it would be helpful if you think about the following and are ready to answer the questions if asked.**
- Your temperature or the temperature of the person you are calling about (if possible).
- Any medicines you or they are taking at the moment.
- Any serious illness you or they have had before.

www.nhsdirect.nhs.uk

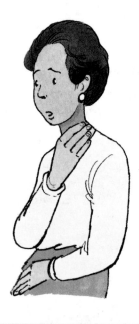

# Sore throat in adults

Has this been going on for more than two weeks or is your voice now hoarse?

 **Yes**

### Call NHS Direct

A long-lasting sore throat, difficulty in swallowing or a hoarse voice needs to be checked by a doctor or nurse. **Speak to your doctor** or call **NHS Direct**.

 **No**

Are your tonsils speckled white or do they have pus on them (the tonsils are the floppy red flaps at each side of the back of the throat, not the single flap hanging down in the middle)?

 **Yes**

### Call NHS Direct

It could be tonsillitis or pharyngitis. Try throat lozenges or gargling with aspirin (not for children under 12). Call **NHS Direct**.

 **No**

Do you have a runny nose and a cough, and are you sneezing?

 **Yes**

### Self-care

It is probably a cold. **Ask your pharmacist** for advice.

 **No**

Are there any tender lumps just below your ear at the angle of your jaw?

 **Yes**

### Self-care

These could be swollen lymph glands which are common with sore throats. Take paracetamol (follow the manufacturer's instructions) to ease the pain.

**No**

*See the opposite page*

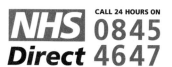
**NHS Direct** CALL 24 HOURS ON **0845 4647**

Do you have a fever, are you feeling flushed, hot and sweaty (is your temperature over 38°C or 100.4°F)?

 **Yes**

## Self-care

If you also have a general feeling of being unwell, a cough and a headache, you probably have a viral infection which will settle on its own. Take paracetamol (follow the manufacturer's instructions).

**No**

Is it impossible to swallow your own saliva?

 **Yes**

## Call NHS Direct

If your throat is so swollen you need medical advice, call **NHS Direct**.

**No**

## Self-care advice

- Drink more fluids – drink something non-alcoholic at least every hour.
- Take regular pain relief, such as paracetamol, following the manufacturer's instructions for correct dosage.
- Avoid foods that cause discomfort when you swallow.
- You can get throat remedies from the pharmacist, who can advise you.
- If new symptoms develop or if your condition worsens, call **NHS Direct**.
- If you are still worried, call **NHS Direct**.

**Before ringing NHS Direct or 999, it would be helpful if you think about the following and are ready to answer the questions if asked.**
- How long you or the person you are calling about have been unwell.
- If you or they are very short of breath or cannot swallow your or their own saliva.
- Your temperature or their temperature (if possible).
- Any medicines you or they are taking at the moment.

www.nhsdirect.nhs.uk

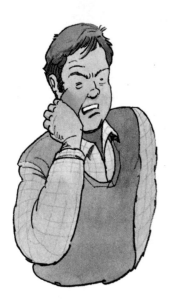

# Toothache

Is the pain severe, continuous and is there no relief with painkillers?

 **Yes**

### Call NHS Direct

You probably have an abscess beneath the tooth. If you have a dentist, call them. If you don't have a dentist, call **NHS Direct** who will be able to help.

 **No**

Does the pain come and go and is it made worse by biting down on the tooth?

 **Yes**

### Self-care

You probably have decay inside one of your teeth. **Make an appointment with your dentist**.

 **No**

Have you recently had a tooth filled by your dentist?

 **Yes**

### Self-care

Pain is common, even for up to a week afterwards. **Ask your pharmacist** for advice. If the pain lasts longer than a week, **call your dentist.**

 **No**

Is there also pain in the front of your face which is made worse with coughing?

 **Yes**

### Call NHS Direct

You may have sinusitis, an infection of the spaces in the bones of the face. Take strong painkillers and ring **NHS Direct**.

**No**

*See the opposite page*

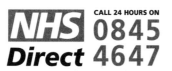

**NHS Direct**  CALL 24 HOURS ON **0845 4647**

**Is there a foul smell in your mouth?**

**Yes**

**No**

### Self-care

Halitosis (smelly breath) can be caused by a number of things, especially food or drink, but a tooth abscess is also a common cause. Do not use breath fresheners or antiseptic mouthwashes too much. **Make an appointment with your dentist.**

### Self-care advice

- Take maximum dose of painkillers, such as paracetamol or ibuprofen, according to the manufacturer's instructions. If you are pregnant, do not take ibuprofen and only take paracetamol as instructed.
- Avoid drinks that are too hot or too cold until your dentist has examined your teeth.
- Avoid food or drinks that contain sugar.
- Contact your dentist as soon as possible.
- If you don't have a dentist, call **NHS Direct** who will be able to help.
- If you are still worried, call **NHS Direct**.

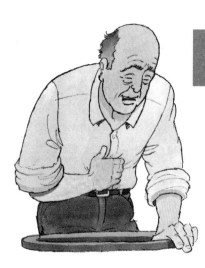

# Vomiting in adults

**Do you have a severe headache?**  Yes

No

### Call NHS Direct

Any severe pain will cause vomiting. If you do not normally suffer from headaches such as migraine, if there has been a recent head injury, or if the light hurts your eyes, you should **dial 999**.

**Has the vomiting been happening regularly over a number of weeks?**  Yes

No

### Self-care

Some women experience frequent vomiting during early pregnancy. Some long-standing conditions like gallstone problems will also cause vomiting. **You can get advice from your pharmacist or doctor**. If you have other symptoms as well as vomiting, you should call **NHS Direct**.

**Do you also have severe abdominal pain which started suddenly?**  Yes

No

If the pain has lasted for more than an hour and is not eased by indigestion remedies (antacids) or by vomiting, call **NHS Direct**.

Go to *Abdominal pain* on page 64 or 72 for more information.

**Is there any blood or brown soil-like material in the vomit?**  Yes

### Call NHS Direct

No

*See the opposite page*

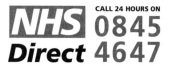

**NHS Direct** CALL 24 HOURS ON **0845 4647**

Do you also have diarrhoea or very loose bowel motions?

**Yes**

**No**

## Self-care

You may have food poisoning. If the vomiting and the diarrhoea are very severe and you are not keeping down fluids or there is blood in the bowel motions, you should call **NHS Direct**. Otherwise take only fluids for at least 12 hours after your symptoms settle, which may take a few days, and **ask your pharmacist's advice**.

## Self-care advice

- Try small amounts of clear fluids or rehydration fluids (for example, Dioralyte) **from your pharmacist**.
- Build up the amount of fluids from sips to a cupful over the next 12 hours.
- 12 hours after the last bout of vomiting, start eating bland foods again (this includes dry biscuits, toast or crackers).
- Avoid milk in your diet during this period.
- Sometimes the cause of vomiting can be a bacterial infection, and can be spread to other people. This means it is important to thoroughly clean all areas that have been in contact with the vomit.
- Be extra careful about personal hygiene, washing hands, and so on.
- Vomiting can make the oral contraceptive pill less effective. Use extra contraception for seven days after your vomiting has stopped and read the information in the pill packet for more advice. Call **NHS Direct** if you are not certain.
- If the condition worsens or new symptoms develop, call **NHS Direct**.
- If you are still worried, call **NHS Direct**.

**Before ringing NHS Direct or 999, it would be helpful if you think about the following and are ready to answer the questions if asked.**
- Your symptoms (the questions you answered 'Yes' to), or the symptoms of the person you are calling about.
- Your temperature or their temperature (if possible).
- When you or they last had anything to eat or drink.
- Any medicines you or they are taking at the moment.
- Any allergies you know of.
- Any serious illnesses you or they have had before.

*Vomiting in adults*

www.nhsdirect.nhs.uk

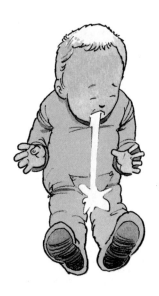

# Vomiting in babies

*Before going through
the following questions, check
'How do I know if my baby is ill?'
on page 5.*

Does the baby have a fever, is the baby flushed, and does it feel hot and sweaty (is the baby's temperature over 38°C or 100.4°F)?

 **Yes**

Go to *Fever in children* on page 30 for more information.

 **No**

Do they have a persistent cough or a runny nose?

 **Yes**

Repeated coughing along with a fever is common with colds and flu and will make the baby vomit. However, there may be other symptoms to look out for.

Go to *Colds and flu* on page 14 for more information.

 **No**

Are there frequent (more than three in 24 hours) watery or very loose bowel motions as well as the vomiting?

 **Yes**

**Call NHS Direct**

 **No**

Is the baby:
– floppy?
– not passing water?
– not taking fluids?

**Yes**

**Call NHS Direct**

Babies can become ill very quickly if they don't have enough fluids.
**Call NHS Direct.**

 **No**

*See the opposite page*

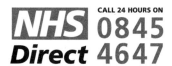

**NHS Direct**  CALL 24 HOURS ON **0845 4647**

Is the vomiting forceful (projectile) and after each feed or is it bile stained (green)?

**Yes**

### Call NHS Direct

There may be a problem with the baby emptying its stomach. Call **NHS Direct**.

**No**

Is the baby crying or moaning continuously or obviously in pain?

**Yes**

### Call NHS Direct

It can be difficult to tell when a baby is in severe pain. If there is a change in the way the baby is crying, particularly if it has been well before, or if there is a rash or fever, call **NHS Direct**.

**No**

Is the vomiting just small amounts after feeds and is the baby otherwise fine?

**Yes**

### Self-care

Babies often bring up small amounts of their feed but it should look similar to their milk feed and should not come out with any force. Winding helps. Using an over-large hole in the teat when bottle-feeding is a common cause. Do not use 'colic treatments' too often.

**No**

### Self-care advice

- If you are breast-feeding, continue as normal, unless vomiting has happened more than twice, in which case call **NHS Direct**.
- If you are bottle-feeding, introduce rehydration fluids (for example, Dioralyte) in small quantities according to the manufacturer's instructions on the pack. Speak to your pharmacist.
- Do not give large amounts of fluids in one go and reintroduce milk gradually.
- If the condition has not improved within two hours or the baby does not have a wet nappy or other symptoms have developed, call **NHS Direct**.
- If you are still worried, call **NHS Direct**.

**Before ringing NHS Direct or 999, it would be helpful if you think about the following and are ready to answer the questions if asked.**
- The symptoms (the questions you answered 'Yes' to).
- Their temperature (if possible).
- When they last had anything to eat or drink.
- Any medicines they are taking at the moment.
- Any allergies you know of.
- Any serious illnesses they have had before.

*Vomiting in babies*

www.nhsdirect.nhs.uk

49

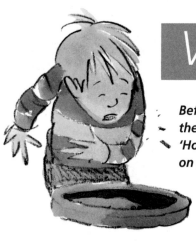

*Before going through the following questions, check 'How do I know if my baby is ill?' on page 5.*

---

**Have they been vomiting for more than one day?**

 **Yes** ▶

### Call NHS Direct

Try just giving fluids rather than solid food but if the child is not taking fluids or is bringing most or all of it up, call **NHS Direct**.

**No** ▼

---

**Do they also have a fever, and is the child flushed, hot and sweaty (is your child's temperature over 38°C or 100.4°F)?**

 **Yes** ▶

### Call NHS Direct

Vomiting is common in children with high temperatures (over 38°C or 100.4°F) and simply lowering their temperature with paracetamol (for example, Calpol) will help.

**Go to *Fever in children* on page 30 for more information.** ▷

**No** ▼

---

**Is the vomit dark brown or does it contain blood?**

 **Yes** ▶

### Call NHS Direct

Vomit in young children should never contain blood or brown soil-like substances. Give them nothing to eat or drink until they have seen a doctor. Call **NHS Direct**.

**No** ▼

---

**Is there severe pain?**

 **Yes** ▶

### Call NHS Direct

Younger children may tuck in their legs and make a moaning sound, particularly after crying continuously for a long time. Call **NHS Direct**.

**Go to *Tummy (abdominal) pain in children* on page 76 for more information.** ▷

**No** ▼

*See the opposite page*

---

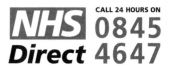

**NHS Direct** CALL 24 HOURS ON **0845 4647**

Do they also have diarrhoea or very loose bowel motions?  **Yes**

### Self-care

It may be gastroenteritis or food poisoning. Call **NHS Direct** if you are not sure.

 **No**

Is your child taking any medicines or tablets?  **Yes**

### Self-care

Occasionally some medicines will cause vomiting. **Ask your pharmacist**. If your child is not able to take any fluids, call **NHS Direct**.

 **No**

Do they have a headache?  **Yes**

A severe headache, such as migraine, can cause vomiting.

Go to *Headache in children* on page 34 for more information.

 **No**

Do they have any pain in their ears?  **Yes**

### Self-care

Infections of the middle ear are common and cause vomiting. If the pain is still there after taking paracetamol (for example, Calpol) **from your pharmacist** for one day, **speak to your doctor**.

 **No**

### Self-care advice

- Give them only sips of water or rehydration fluids (for example, Dioralyte – your pharmacist can advise) for the first two hours.
- Gradually increase the amount of clear fluids or rehydration fluids they have every two hours.
- Build up to a bland diet after eight hours (for example, avoid fatty or spicy foods).
- If the condition gets worse or other symptoms develop, call **NHS Direct**.
- If you are still worried, call **NHS Direct**.

**Before ringing NHS Direct or 999, it would be helpful if you think about the following and are ready to answer the questions if asked.**
- Their symptoms (the questions you answered 'Yes' to).
- Their temperature (if possible).
- When they last had anything to eat or drink.
- Any medicines they are taking at the moment.
- Any allergies you know of.
- Any serious illnesses they have had before.

*Vomiting in children*

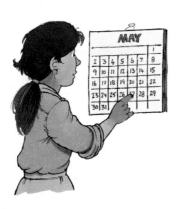

# Absent periods

Do you normally bleed after sex, which is not related to your period?

 **Yes**

### Call NHS Direct

Any bleeding, other than during your period, should be checked.

Go to *Adult vaginal bleeding* on page 54 for more information.

**No**

Could you be pregnant?

 **Yes**

### Self-care

**See your pharmacist**. Check if you are pregnant by using a home testing kit. If you are unsure, call **NHS Direct**.

**No**

Have you recently given birth?

 **Yes**

### Self-care

Although all women are different, periods will often be delayed by at least six months after childbirth. Breast-feeding can make this delay longer but you can still become pregnant again during this time.

Have there been any major events in your life, such as a bereavement, family illness or moving house?

 **Yes**

### Call NHS Direct

Hormones do change when you have been stressed and this can cause irregular periods.

**No**

Have you lost weight over the past few months, either intentionally or for no apparent reason?

 **Yes**

### Call NHS Direct

Losing weight too quickly by dieting can cause a delay in your periods. If you are concerned about someone who has lost too much weight, call **NHS Direct** or **speak to your doctor**. If the weight loss was not deliberate, you should call **NHS Direct**.

See *Weight loss* on page 123 for more information.

**No**

*See the opposite page*

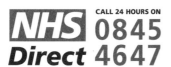

**NHS Direct** CALL 24 HOURS ON **0845 4647**

Did you recently stop taking oral contraceptives (the pill)?

**Yes**

### Self-care

Depending on the type of contraceptive pill, it can take several months before normal periods start again.

See *Contraception* on page 116 for more information.

**No**

---

Are you getting close to the menopause or are you over 45?

**Yes**

### Self-care

As you get closer to the menopause, your periods may become irregular before they stop completely.

See *Menopause* on page 105 for more information.

**No**

---

Has there been any change in your activity, weight, hairiness or voice?

**Yes**

### Call NHS Direct

Changes in hormones, such as thyroxine, can produce these changes and can also make your periods irregular.

**No**

---

Are you taking any medicines?

**Yes**

### Call NHS Direct

Some medicines and herbal treatments can change the pattern of your periods. **Ask your pharmacist** or call **NHS Direct**.

**No**

---

### Self-care advice

- Although it can be very worrying, if you are otherwise fit and well, a missed period alone will not need urgent medical attention.
- Make sure you have a well-balanced diet and take regular normal exercise. This is important to stay fit and healthy.
- Keep an accurate diary of your menstrual cycle (periods). It will be helpful if you need to get more advice.
- If the condition gets worse or new symptoms develop, call **NHS Direct**.
- If you are still worried or need further help, call **NHS Direct**.

---

Before ringing **NHS Direct** or 999, it would be helpful if you think about the following and are ready to answer the questions if asked.
- Where the pain is.
- Any previous pregnancies.
- The date of your last period (or that of the person you are calling about).
- Information on the contraception you or they use.
- If you or they have had a pregnancy test – when and what the result was.
- The results of your or their last cervical smear.
- Your or their temperature (if possible).

# *Adult vaginal bleeding*

Are you pregnant and registered with a midwife?  **Yes**

### Self-care

**Speak to your midwife**.

 **No**

Could you be pregnant?  **Yes**

### Call NHS Direct

Vaginal bleeding during pregnancy does happen without any harm to either baby or mother, but it should always be checked with **NHS Direct** as it can be serious.

 **No**

Did your periods stop more than three months ago?  **Yes**

### Call NHS Direct

Even if your pregnancy test was negative, you might still be pregnant. If you have passed the menopause, it could show something is wrong with your cervix or womb. You should call **NHS Direct** immediately.

 **No**

Does the bleeding only happen after sex?  **Yes**

### Call NHS Direct

If you have not had a cervical smear performed within the past year or are waiting for results from a recent test, you should call **NHS Direct** for advice.

 **No**

*See the opposite page*

**NHS Direct** CALL 24 HOURS ON **0845 4647**

Are you taking an oral contraceptive and have changed the type recently?

**Yes**

### Call NHS Direct

Breakthrough bleeding is common especially if you have recently changed your oral contraceptive pill or if you have been ill, are vomiting or have diarrhoea. If it continues, see your family planning advisor or your doctor. Call **NHS Direct**.

**No**

Have you only just started having periods within the past three years?

**Yes**

### Call NHS Direct

Irregular periods are very common to begin with. If they continue to be irregular, call **NHS Direct**.

**No**

Do you think you have started or are getting close to the menopause?

**Yes**

### Call NHS Direct

Periods often become irregular as you get close to the menopause, but there should never be any bleeding after you have been through the menopause.
If there is bleeding, call **NHS Direct**.

**No**

Do you have severe pain, do you have an intrauterine contraceptive device (coil) or are you pregnant?

**Yes**

### Call NHS Direct

There is a possibility of a pregnancy outside the normal place within the womb. This is a greater possibility if you have ever had a serious infection of the womb or if you have had a sterilisation reversed. Call **NHS Direct**.

**No**

### Self-care advice

- Try resting and keep a record of the sanitary towels or tampons you use. This will help to assess the amount of blood you lose.
- Take painkillers, such as paracetamol, if you have pain or discomfort.
- You will need to book a routine appointment with your GP if this is happening regularly.
- If any new symptoms develop or the condition worsens, call **NHS Direct**.
- If you are still worried, call **NHS Direct**.

**Before ringing NHS Direct or 999, it would be helpful if you think about the following and are ready to answer the questions if asked.**
- Where the pain is.
- Any previous pregnancies.
- The date of your last period (or that of the person you are calling about).
- Information on the contraception you or they use.
- If you or they have had a pregnancy test – when and what the result was.
- Results of your or their last cervical smear.
- Your or their temperature (if possible).

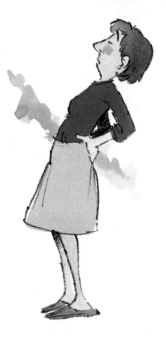

# Backache in adults

Do you have one or more of the following symptoms?
- Numbness and tingling in your limbs.
- Difficulty moving your limbs.
- No control over your water or bowel motions.

 **Yes**  **Call NHS Direct**

 **No**

Does the pain travel down the back of one or both legs?

 **Yes**  **Call NHS Direct**

You may have pressure on the sciatic nerve. Call **NHS Direct**.

 **No**

Do you also have a fever, are you feeling flushed, hot and sweaty (is your temperature over 38°C or 100.4°F)?

 **Yes**  **Call NHS Direct**

 **No**

Does the pain move from the middle of your back to your groin?

 **Yes**  **Call NHS Direct**

 **No**

Did the pain start suddenly, for example after a fall?

 **Yes**  **Self-care**

Most back pain after an injury is simply bruising or strained soft tissue, such as ligament or muscle, and can be helped with paracetamol or anti-inflammatory medicines. **Ask your pharmacist**.

**No**

*See the opposite page*

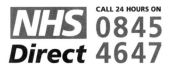
**NHS** CALL 24 HOURS ON **0845**
**Direct 4647**

Did the pain start after
lifting a heavy weight?

**Yes**

### Self-care

If the pain is only at one point in your
back, you have probably strained a ligament
or muscle and **do not need to speak
to your doctor**. Paracetamol and
anti-inflammatory medicines, such as
ibuprofen, will help. Do not stay in bed, but
take gentle exercise until the pain eases.

**No**

Is the pain worse after sitting
for a long time?

**Yes**

### Self-care

Your posture may be wrong and
simple painkillers will help.
**Ask your pharmacist** for advice.

**No**

Is the pain tearing or ripping?

**Yes**

### Call NHS Direct

**No**

### Self-care advice

- Do not do any lifting, but gentle
  stretching exercises may help.
- Try simple painkillers, such as
  paracetamol, or your usual
  pain relief.
- Avoid medication that contains
  codeine as it may cause constipation.
- Try applying heat packs or ice packs
  to the area, for no longer than
  five minutes at a time. Repeat every
  hour. You should wrap ice packs
  in a tea towel to avoid any contact
  with the skin.
- If the condition gets worse or new
  symptoms develop, call **NHS Direct**.
- If you are still worried, call
  **NHS Direct**.

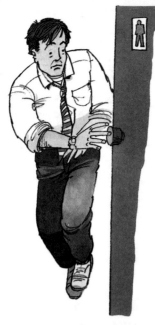

# Diarrhoea in adults

Is there any red blood in the diarrhoea or severe tummy (abdominal) pain?

 **Yes**

### Call NHS Direct

If there is a large amount of blood or tar-like material in the bowel motions, **dial 999**.

 **No**

Have you had persistent diarrhoea for more than a few weeks?

 **Yes**

### Call NHS Direct

 **No**

Are you taking any medicines at the moment?

 **Yes**

### Self-care

Some medicines, such as antibiotics, can cause diarrhoea. **Ask your pharmacist** for advice.

 **No**

Are you also vomiting or are any other members of your family or any friends also affected, who may have eaten similar food within the past three days?

 **Yes**

### Self-care

You may have gastroenteritis or food poisoning. If it is very mild, avoid solid food and milk for a day and drink only non-alcoholic fluids. **Your pharmacist will advise you** about medicines to stop diarrhoea. If it is severe or there is also pain, or blood in your bowel motions, call **NHS Direct**.

 **No**

*See the opposite page*

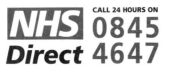

**NHS** CALL 24 HOURS ON
**Direct** 0845
4647

## Self-care advice

- Drink clear fluids only for 24 hours, for example, water.
- Oral rehydration fluids (for example, Dioralyte) are available **from your pharmacist** and may help.
- Introduce soft, bland foods, such as potatoes, bread and dry biscuits, in small amounts.
- Once your bowel motions are more solid, you can start eating your usual diet.
- Avoid fruit and foods that contain roughage, such as bran, until your diarrhoea has stopped.
- Diarrhoea can make the oral contraceptive pill less effective. Use extra contraception for seven days after your diarrhoea has stopped, and read the information in the pill packet for more advice. Call **NHS Direct** if you are not certain.
- If the condition gets worse or new symptoms develop, call **NHS Direct**.
- If you are still worried, call **NHS Direct**.

**Before ringing NHS Direct or 999, it would be helpful if you think about the following and are ready to answer the questions if asked.**

- Your or their symptoms (the questions you answered 'Yes' to), or the symptoms of the person you are calling about.
- If you or they have travelled abroad recently.
- Your temperature or their temperature (if possible).
- When you or they last had anything to eat or drink.
- Any medicines you or they are taking at the moment.
- Any allergies you know of.
- Any serious illnesses you or they have had before.

*Diarrhoea in adults*

www.nhsdirect.nhs.uk

# Diarrhoea in babies and children

*Before going through the following questions, check 'How do I know if my baby is ill?' on page 5.*

Has your baby had watery or very loose bowel motions more than three times in the last 24 hours?

 **Yes**    **Call NHS Direct**

 **No**

Does the baby have a fever, is the baby flushed, hot and sweaty (is the baby's temperature over 38°C or 100.4°F)?

 **Yes**    **Call NHS Direct**

 **No**

Is your baby also vomiting and not keeping fluids down?

 **Yes**    **Call NHS Direct**

 **No**

Is there blood in the diarrhoea?

 **Yes**    **Call NHS Direct**

 **No**

Are you adding sugar to fruit juices or the bottle feeds?

 **Yes**    **Self-care**

Sugar may cause diarrhoea and make existing diarrhoea worse. **Ask your health visitor** for advice.

 **No**

Has your baby just started solid foods?

 **Yes**    **Self-care**

It may be too soon for solid foods. **Ask your health visitor** for advice.

 **No**

*See the opposite page*

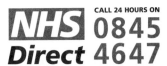

**NHS** CALL 24 HOURS ON **0845**
**Direct** **4647**

**Has your baby just started taking new medicines?**

**Yes**

## Self-care ✚

Some medicines, such as antibiotics, can cause diarrhoea. Do not stop the medicines. **Ask your pharmacist** for advice.

**No**

## Self-care advice ✚

- Watery or very loose bowel motions are common in babies and young children. If the baby is otherwise well, it is likely that the diarrhoea will settle within 24 hours.
- It depends how thirsty the baby or child is as to how much fluid they need.
- *For breast-fed babies:*
  – Continue to feed them when they need it.
  – You can also give them extra drinks or rehydration fluids (for example, Dioralyte) between feeds.
  – For more detailed advice, **ask your health visitor**.
- *For bottle-fed babies:*
  – Offer as much fluids or oral rehydration fluids (for example, Dioralyte) as your baby needs for the first four hours.
  – If their diarrhoea continues, switch between the bottle feed and oral rehydration fluids for the next eight hours.
  – Then introduce normal feeds.
  – For more detailed advice, **ask your health visitor**.
- *For older children:*
  – Avoid giving them solid foods until the child's appetite has returned.
  – Offer as much fluid as the child needs (avoid cow's milk for 24 hours until the diarrhoea settles down).
  – Oral rehydration fluids (for example, Dioralyte) will also help. You can get these **from your pharmacist**.
- If any new symptoms develop or the condition gets worse, call **NHS Direct**.
- If you are still worried, call **NHS Direct**.

**Before ringing NHS Direct or 999, it would be helpful if you think about the following and are ready to answer the questions if asked.**
- Their symptoms (the questions you answered 'Yes' to).
- Their temperature (if possible).
- When they last had anything to eat or drink.
- Any medicines they are taking at the moment.
- Any allergies you know of.
- Any serious illnesses they have had before.

*Diarrhoea in babies and children*

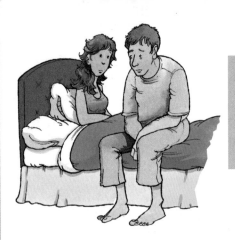

## Erectile problems and impotence

Do you suffer from diabetes, hypertension (high blood pressure), hardened arteries or damage to the nervous system, for example, multiple sclerosis?

 **Yes**

**Call NHS Direct**

These conditions can affect the ability to get and maintain an erection but may be treated by your doctor.

 **No**

Have you damaged your spine in an accident or through disease?

 **Yes**

**Call NHS Direct**

Injury or disease of the nerves in the spine can cause problems with getting an erection. It is possible to overcome this through various treatments.

 **No**

Are you on any medication?

 **Yes**

**Call NHS Direct**

Some medicines, such as beta-blockers and antidepressants, can cause erectile dysfunction (problems getting an erection). Do not stop taking them before you find out whether there is a suitable alternative.

 **No**

Are you very anxious, very stressed or depressed?

 **Yes**

**Call NHS Direct**

Your mental state can have a major influence over your ability to get an erection. Dealing with the cause of the stress or anxiety can often lead to an improvement. Depression can also be treated by your doctor. Call **NHS Direct**.

 **No**

Are you regularly drinking heavily?

 **Yes**

**Call NHS Direct**

Too much alcohol will affect getting an erection. As regular alcohol abuse causes high blood pressure, this will also affect erections.

 **No**

*See the opposite page*

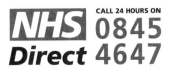

CALL 24 HOURS ON
**NHS** 0845
*Direct* 4647

Do you smoke?  **Yes**

### Call NHS Direct

 **No**

Nicotine and carbon monoxide from tobacco affect erections both immediately and in the longer term. Cigarettes cause hardened arteries, which lead to problems with erections. If you'd like help to stop smoking, call the NHS Smoking Helpline on **0800 1690169**.

See *Smoking and lung cancer* on page 112 for more information.

---

Do you and your partner have little chance of being alone while making love?  **Yes**

### Self-care

Anxiety over interruption can affect erections, but this can be treated by dealing with the anxiety.

 **No**

---

Are you experiencing relationship difficulties or having an affair with someone else?  **Yes**

### Self-care

Feelings of guilt or lack of attraction can cause a failure of erection, but this is not a disease and will not respond to medical treatment.

 **No**

---

Do you have erections during the night (does your partner notice or do you wake up with an erection)?  **Yes**

### Self-care

You do not have erectile dysfunction and your problem is probably related to your relationship, stress or dissatisfaction rather than to a disease.

 **No**

---

### Self-care advice

- Most erection problems are caused by psychological factors such as stress and anxiety.
- Try to avoid drinking too much alcohol or smoking.
- Make sure the environment is right and that you're unlikely to be disturbed.
- If the condition gets worse or new symptoms develop, call **NHS Direct**.
- If you are still worried, call **NHS Direct**.

**Before ringing NHS Direct or 999, it would be helpful if you think about the following and are ready to answer the questions if asked.**
- Any medicines you or the person you are calling about are taking at the moment.
- Any serious illness you or they have had before.

www.nhsdirect.nhs.uk

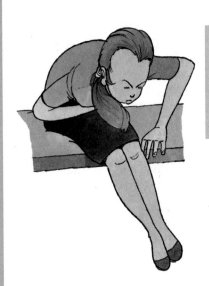

# Female abdominal pain in adults

Is the pain just below your ribcage or in the upper part of the tummy, extending into the chest, is it crushing, does it last more than 15 minutes and is it not eased by indigestion remedies?  **Yes** **Dial 999**

 **No**

Is your period late or do you have unusual bleeding? Could you be pregnant?  **Yes** **Call NHS Direct**

 **No**

Have you felt a similar pain more than once over the past few weeks?  **Yes** Go to *Long-standing abdominal pain* on page 70 for more information.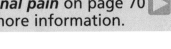

 **No**

Is the pain severe and have you a swollen tummy or fever or vomiting?  **Yes** **Call NHS Direct**

 **No**

Is there a lot of blood or soil-like material in the vomit?  **Yes** **Call NHS Direct**

 **No**

*See the opposite page*

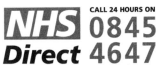

**NHS Direct** CALL 24 HOURS ON **0845 4647**

Is there tar-like material or blood in the bowel motions? **Yes**  → **Call NHS Direct**

 **No**

Is the pain also moving to your groin? **Yes**  → **Call NHS Direct**

You may have an infection of the kidney or a kidney stone. If there is no relief with paracetamol or the pain is very severe, call **NHS Direct**.

Go to *Female urinary and vaginal problems in adults* on page 68 for more information.

 **No**

Do you have diarrhoea? **Yes**  → **Self-care**

Diarrhoea can be caused by some medicines such as antibiotics. **Ask your pharmacist** about any medicines you are taking. If there is also severe pain or vomiting, it may mean food poisoning. Call **NHS Direct**.

Go to *Diarrhoea in adults* on page 58 for more information.

 **No**

Has it been a few days since your last bowel motion? **Yes**  → **Self-care**

Some medicines can cause constipation, especially painkillers. **Ask your pharmacist** about any medicines you are taking. If there is severe pain or tummy (abdominal) swelling, or vomiting, or it has lasted for more than a few days, call **NHS Direct**.

**No**

Is there a tender, tingling sensation along with the pain on only one side of the tummy? **Yes** → **Call NHS Direct**

You may have shingles. If this is your first attack of shingles, you should call **NHS Direct**. If you have frequent attacks of shingles, **speak to your doctor**.

Go to *Shingles* on page 111 for more information.

**No**

*See the next page*

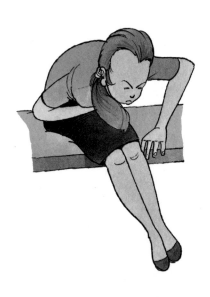

## Female abdominal pain in adults, continued

Are you passing blood from your vagina even though it is not time for your period?

 **Yes**

You should report any bleeding from the vagina, either between periods or especially after the menopause, to your doctor.

 Go to *Adult vaginal bleeding* on page 54 for more information.

 **No**

Do you have discharge from your vagina which is different from the usual or which may be smelly?

 **Yes**

**Call NHS Direct**

Tell **NHS Direct** you have a severe lower abdominal pain. Tell them your temperature, any medicines you are on, any allergies, if you are pregnant, and details of any contraception you are taking.

 **No**

Does it sting badly when you pass water?

 **Yes**

**Self-care**

Cystitis (bladder infection) can be eased by a covered hot-water bottle, plenty of fluids and paracetamol. If it is not settling with the use of over-the-counter medicines, **see your doctor**.

Go to *Cystitis* on page 94 for more information.

**No**

Is it happening at the same time as your period?

 **Yes**

**Ask your pharmacist**

Period pain can be severe for some women and can happen for the first time after many years of painless periods. Try a hot-water bottle against your tummy at night or when you are sitting down. Anti-inflammatory medicines can help. **Ask your pharmacist** for advice.

**No**

*See the opposite page*

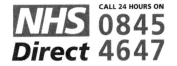

**NHS** CALL 24 HOURS ON
**Direct** **0845 4647**

## Self-care advice

- Try to relieve the pain by resting.
- If you are not vomiting, try taking simple painkillers.
- If the condition gets worse or new symptoms develop, call **NHS Direct**.
- If you are still worried, call **NHS Direct**.

**Before ringing NHS Direct or 999, it would be helpful if you think about the following and are ready to answer the questions if asked.**

- How long you or the person you are calling about have been unwell.
- If it may be a heart attack.
- If you or they are pregnant.
- If there is any vaginal bleeding.
- If the tummy (abdomen) is very tender and swollen.
- If there is any blood, tar or soil-like material in the vomit or bowel motions.
- If the pain is in the back, moving down to the groin.
- Your temperature or their temperature (if possible).
- If there is anyone else in the house with the same problem.
- When you or they last had anything to eat or drink.
- Any medicines you or they are taking at the moment.
- Any illnesses, such as bowel, heart, stomach or kidney problems, that you or they have had before.

www.nhsdirect.nhs.uk

# Female urinary and vaginal problems in adults

*For* adult vaginal bleeding, *see page 54.*

| | | |
|---|---|---|
| Are you passing blood in your water? |  **Yes** | **Call NHS Direct**  |
|  **No** | | |
| Is there a smelly, green or yellow vaginal discharge or itchiness? |  **Yes** | **Call NHS Direct**  |
|  **No** | | |
| Do you have a fever, are you feeling flushed, hot and sweaty (is your temperature over 38°C or 100.4°F), are there brown blood clots in your urine and do you have a severe pain in your lower back? |  **Yes** | **Call NHS Direct**  |
|  **No** | | |

Are you passing water more often than usual and does it sting each time?     **Yes**

**Self-care**

You may have a bladder (water) infection (cystitis). Drink plenty of fluids and take paracetamol. If there is no improvement after two days, call **NHS Direct**.

Go to *Cystitis* on page 94 for more information.

 **No**

*See the opposite page*

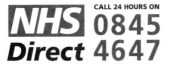

**NHS** CALL 24 HOURS ON
**Direct** 0845 4647

Is there a creamy white vaginal discharge or itchiness?

**Yes**

**No**

### Self-care

You may have thrush (Candida). **See your pharmacist**. If you have repeated attacks over a short space of time, call **NHS Direct**.

Go to *Vaginal thrush* on page 115 for more information.

Are you also experiencing vaginal bleeding?

**Yes**

**No**

Go to *Adult vaginal bleeding* on page 54 for more information.

### Self-care advice

- Avoid sexual intercourse until the problem is sorted out.
- Increase how much you drink to at least eight glasses of fluid a day. Juices such as barley water and cranberry may help.
- Over-the-counter medicines **from your pharmacist** may also help. They will be able to advise you.
- Avoid using soap for bathing as this can cause irritation. Take showers if possible.
- Keep an eye on the area around the vagina for signs of soreness, in which case call **NHS Direct**.
- If new symptoms develop or if your condition worsens, call **NHS Direct**.
- If you are still worried, call **NHS Direct**.

**Before ringing NHS Direct or 999, it would be helpful if you think about the following and are ready to answer the questions if asked.**
- How long you or the person you are calling about have been unwell.
- Your or their temperature (if possible).
- If there is severe back pain which moves to the groin.
- Any medicines you or they are taking at the moment.

# Long-standing abdominal pain in adults

Is your appetite poor or have you lost weight over the past two months for no apparent reason?

 **Yes**

 **No**

### Call NHS Direct

If the symptoms are not getting better with indigestion remedies, call **NHS Direct**.

Is the pain a burning sensation deep inside the upper tummy, which is made worse when you lie down or bend over?

 **Yes**

 **No**

### Self-care

You may have stomach acid leaking into the gullet, which is common and is treatable with indigestion remedies (antacids) or medicines which block the production of stomach acid or make the stomach move its contents on quicker. You should use an extra pillow at night and avoid foods that bring on the pain. **Ask your pharmacist** for advice.
If the pain is severe or your bowel motions are black and like tar, you should call **NHS Direct**.

Go to *Hiatus hernia* on page 98 for more information.

Is the pain relieved by drinking milk or taking indigestion remedies (antacids)?

 **Yes**

 **No**

*See the opposite page*

### Self-care

Inflammation of the stomach wall (gastritis) is quite common, particularly after rich food or alcohol. It should settle with simple indigestion remedies. **Ask your pharmacist** for advice.
If the pain is severe or you are passing bowel motions that are black and like tar or are vomiting soil-like material, call **NHS Direct**.

Go to *Indigestion* on page 99 and *Peptic ulcers* on page 108 for more information.

**NHS Direct**
CALL 24 HOURS ON
**0845 4647**

Is the pain on the right side just under your ribs and is your temperature raised?

**Yes**

 **No**

## Self-care

Avoid those foods, usually fatty meals, which trigger the pain. Take paracetamol for the pain, avoid all food, and drink only water until the pain goes away. If the problem continues, you may become jaundiced with a yellow tinge to your skin and the whites of your eyes. **In these circumstances you should call NHS Direct**. If you have not been diagnosed as having gallstone problems by your doctor, you should make an appointment.

Do you get tummy bloating and have irregular bowel motions?

**Yes**

 **No**

## Self-care advice

- Try resting.
- If you are not vomiting, take fluids in small quantities only for the next 12 hours.
- Take simple painkillers such as paracetamol (do not take aspirin or codeine).
- If the condition gets worse or other symptoms develop, call **NHS Direct**.
- If you are still worried, call **NHS Direct**.

## Self-care

You may have irritable bowel syndrome (IBS) which is common but not serious. Avoiding those things which make it worse, such as certain foods, stress and so on, is important. You should **see your doctor** if:
– the home treatment doesn't work after two weeks;
– you pass blood in your motions;
– your bowel motions are very dark, black or covered with mucus; or
– there is an unexplained weight loss.

Go to *Irritable bowel syndrome* on page 100 for more information.

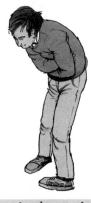

# Male abdominal pain in adults

Is the pain just below your ribcage or in the upper part of your tummy, extending into the chest, is it crushing, does it last more than 15 minutes and is it not eased by indigestion remedies?

 **Yes** ▶ **Dial 999**

 **No**

Is there a severe pain in one of your testicles which started very suddenly?

 **Yes** ▶ **Call NHS Direct**

 **No**

Have you felt a similar pain more than once over the past few weeks?

 **Yes** ▶ Go to *Long-standing abdominal pain* on page 70 for more information.

 **No**

Is the pain severe and do you have a swollen tummy (visibly big and tight) or fever or vomiting?

 **Yes** ▶ **Call NHS Direct**

 **No**

Is there a lot of blood or soil-like material in the vomit?

 **Yes** ▶ **Call NHS Direct**

 **No**

Is there tar-like material or blood in the bowel motions?

 **Yes** ▶ **Call NHS Direct**

 **No**

*See the opposite page*

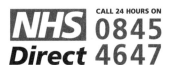 **CALL 24 HOURS ON** **0845 4647**

Is there a tender, tingling sensation along with the pain on only one side of the tummy?

**Yes** ▶

### Call NHS Direct

You may have shingles. If this is your first attack of shingles, you should call **NHS Direct**. If you are having repeated attacks of shingles, you should **tell your doctor**.

Go to *Shingles* on page 111 for more information. ▶

**No** ▼

As well as the pain, are there frequent bouts of diarrhoea?

**Yes** ▶

### Self-care

Diarrhoea can be caused by medicines such as antibiotics. **Ask your pharmacist** about any medicines you are taking. If there is also severe pain or vomiting (or both), it may mean food poisoning. Call **NHS Direct**.

◀ Go to *Diarrhoea in adults* on page 58 for more information.

**No** ▼

Is the pain also moving to your groin?

**Yes** ▶

### Call NHS Direct

You may have an infection of the kidney or a kidney stone. If there is no relief with paracetamol or the pain is very severe, call **NHS Direct**.

Go to *Male urinary and penile problems in adults* on page 74 for more information. ▶

**No** ▼

Has it been a few days since your last bowel motion?

**Yes** ▶

### Self-care

Some medicines, especially painkillers, will cause constipation. **Ask your pharmacist** about any medicines you are taking. If there is severe pain or tummy (abdominal) swelling, or vomiting, or it has lasted for more than a few days, **speak to your doctor**.

**No** ▼

### Self-care advice

- Try to relieve the pain by resting.
- If you are not vomiting, try taking simple painkillers.
- Watch closely for signs of restlessness or the condition becoming worse – in which case call **NHS Direct**.
- If new symptoms develop or the pain gets worse, call **NHS Direct**.
- If you are still worried, call **NHS Direct**.

**Before ringing NHS Direct or 999, it would be helpful if you think about the following and are ready to answer the questions if asked.**
- How long you or the person you are calling about have been unwell.
- If it may be a heart attack.
- If the tummy (abdomen) is very tender and swollen.
- If there is any blood, tar or soil-like material in the vomit or bowel motions.
- If the pain is in the back moving down the groin.
- Your temperature or their temperature (if possible).
- If there is anyone else in the house with the same problem.
- When you or they last had anything to eat or drink.
- Any medicines you or they are taking at the moment.
- Any illnesses, such as bowel, heart, stomach or kidney problems, you or they have had before.

# Male urinary and penile problems in adults

Is there a severe pain in one of your testicles which started suddenly?

**Yes** ▶ **Call NHS Direct**

 **No**

Is there a discharge from the penis?

**Yes** ▶ **Call NHS Direct**

You may have an infection. Either call **NHS Direct** or go to your local genito-urinary clinic where you do not have to give your name.

 **No**

Is there a heavy, dull, dragging pain in your groin with a fever, are you feeling flushed, hot and sweaty (is your temperature over 38°C or 100.4°F)?

**Yes** ▶ **Call NHS Direct**

 **No**

Is it painful to urinate and are you passing water much more often than usual?

**Yes** ▶ **Call NHS Direct**

Drink plenty of fluids and call **NHS Direct**.

 **No**

*See the opposite page*

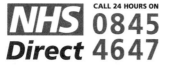 **CALL 24 HOURS ON 0845 4647**

Are you over 45, is your urine stream weak and do you have to pass water very often, even during the night?  **Yes**  **Call NHS Direct**

 **No**

Is there any blood in your urine?  **Yes** **Call NHS Direct**

 **No**

Is there any blood in your sperm?  **Yes** **Call NHS Direct**

 **No**

## Self-care advice

General advice for urinary problems.

- Avoid sexual intercourse until the problem is sorted out.
- Increase how much you drink to at least eight glasses of fluid a day. Juices such as barley water or cranberry may help.
- Over-the-counter medicines **from your pharmacist** may also help. They will be able to advise you.
- Avoid using soap for bathing as this can cause irritation. Take showers if possible.
- Watch out for signs of soreness around the penis, in which case call **NHS Direct**.
- If new symptoms develop or if your condition worsens, call **NHS Direct**.
- If you are still worried, call **NHS Direct**.

**Before ringing NHS Direct or 999, it would be helpful if you think about the following and are ready to answer the questions if asked.**

- Your symptoms (the questions you answered 'Yes' to), or the symptoms of the person you are calling about.
- Your temperature or their temperature (if possible).
- When you or they last had anything to eat or drink.
- Any medicines you or they are taking at the moment.
- Any allergies you know of.
- Any serious illnesses you or they have had before.

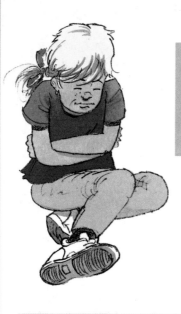

# Tummy (abdominal) pain in children

*Before going through
the following questions, check
'How do I know if my baby is ill?'
on page 5.*

If the child is male, is there a severe pain in one of his testicles which started very suddenly?

 **Call NHS Direct**

 **No**

Is it painful for them to pass water or are they passing water much more often than usual?

 **Call NHS Direct**

They may have a bladder (water) infection. Call **NHS Direct** for advice.

 **No**

Do they have a fever, are they flushed, hot and sweaty (is their temperature over 38°C or 100.4°F) and are they vomiting and not able to keep down any fluids?

 **Call NHS Direct**

Children rapidly dehydrate when they have a fever and they cannot take fluids due to vomiting. Call **NHS Direct**.

 **No**

Is there any blood in their vomit or bowel motions?

 **Call NHS Direct**

 **No**

Is the child screaming constantly or vomiting, and does movement of any kind make it worse?

 **Call NHS Direct**

 **No**

*See the opposite page*

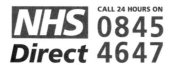

**NHS** CALL 24 HOURS ON **0845**
**Direct** **4647**

Has your child accidentally taken some tablets or medicines, or eaten poisonous plants, such as laburnum seeds?

**Yes**

**Call NHS Direct**

**No**

Has your child just eaten a large amount of fruit or foods they do not usually eat?

**Yes**

**Self-care**

Overeating, especially of acidic fruit, can cause tummy pain. Try simple indigestion remedies like milk. If the symptoms don't improve or they worsen or there are any other symptoms within 24 hours, call **NHS Direct**.

**No**

Is your child constipated?

**Yes**

**Self-care**

Not enough fluids, particularly in hot weather, can cause constipation in children. If the symptoms don't improve or if they develop a new symptom such as vomiting, call **NHS Direct**. Otherwise **ask your pharmacist** for advice.

**No**

Does the tummy pain only start before they are about to go to school or after they come home?

**Yes**

**Self-care**

It could be stress or anxiety about school or the pressure of homework. A chat about it with their teacher may help. In the short term, paracetamol (for example, Calpol) may ease the symptoms but you should not use it regularly.

**No**

### Self-care advice

- Reassure the child and try to help them rest.
- Tummy pain in children is common and normally gets better within 24 hours.
- If they are not being sick, try giving them paracetamol (for example, Calpol) (follow the instructions on the packet to make sure you give the correct dose for your child's age).
- Give them only small amounts of clear fluids for 12 hours, then small amounts of their usual food (without milk) until the child feels better.
- If the condition gets worse or new symptoms develop, call **NHS Direct**.
- If you are still worried, call **NHS Direct**.

Before ringing **NHS Direct** or **999**, it would be helpful if you think about the following and are ready to answer the questions if asked.
- How long they have been unwell.
- If the tummy (abdomen) is very tender and swollen.
- If there is any blood, tar-like or soil-like material in the vomit or bowel motions.
- Their temperature (if possible).
- If there is anyone else in the house with the same problem.
- When they last had anything to eat or drink.
- Any medicines they are taking at the moment.

*Tummy (abdominal) pain in children*

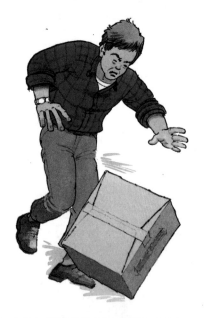

# Injuries to hands and feet

*The advice is suitable for adults and children.*

Have you lost a limb,
a finger or a toe?

 **Yes**

## Dial 999

- Press on the wound with a clean cloth or bandage to stop you losing blood.
- Lift the hand or foot higher than waist height.
- If possible, lie the person down and lift the foot or hand higher than their chest.
- Put the finger or toe into a plastic bag.
- Put this bag into another bag containing ice.
- Do not let the ice come into direct contact with the finger or toe.
- Take this with you to your local hospital's accident and emergency department and tell the ambulance crew what you have done. It may be possible to sew it back on.

 **No**

Is it very difficult or impossible
to move any fingers, toes, feet
or hands?

 **Yes**

## Call NHS Direct

You may have broken a bone, dislocated a joint or damaged a tendon.

 **No**

Have your fingernails or toenails
been crushed and is there a blue
colour under your nail, along with
a throbbing pain?

 **Yes**

## Call NHS Direct

There is probably blood trapped under the nail. It is possible to release this blood but if it is not too painful, it will settle on its own. Sometimes the nail will come away. It takes around six months for a new nail to completely grow back. Call **NHS Direct**.

 **No**

*See the opposite page*

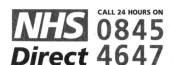

**NHS** CALL 24 HOURS ON
**Direct** 0845 4647

Is there a gaping wound
which is still bleeding?

 **Yes**

## Call NHS Direct

You may need to have the wound stitched.

 **No**

Is the cut minor and is it easy to
stop the blood from flowing?

 **Yes**

## Self-care

Clean the wound with tap water and cover
with an adhesive plaster or dry bandage. If
the person is not protected against tetanus,
they should contact their GP's surgery.

 **No**

## Call NHS Direct

If you cannot sort out what to do
from this list, please call **NHS Direct**.

**Before ringing NHS Direct or 999, it
would be helpful if you think about
the following and are ready to answer
the questions if asked.**

■ If there is a serious wound with loss
of blood.
■ If there is a serious crush injury and
you or the person you are calling
about cannot move their fingers or
toes.
■ If any fingers or toes have been
completely torn off.
■ If any bones are sticking out of
the wound.

*Injuries to hands and feet*

www.nhsdirect.nhs.uk

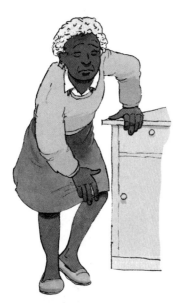

# Joint pains

*This advice is suitable for adults. Joint pain in children is not common but when it happens, you should get advice from **NHS Direct**.*

Does the joint have an unusual appearance and is it difficult or impossible to move?

 **Call NHS Direct**

You may have dislocated or broken the joint. Call **NHS Direct**.

**No**

Did the pain start suddenly after an accident or exercise?

 **Self-care**

Most joint injuries are sprains and only need the following.
**Rest**: Stop using the joint until the pain eases.
**Ice**: Use ice or frozen peas in a cloth cover for no more than five minutes. Never allow direct contact with the skin.
**Elevation**: If possible, lift and support the limb to reduce swelling.

 Go to *Injuries to hands and feet* on page 78 for more information.

**No**

Do you have any of the following symptoms?
– Severe pain.
– The joint is very hot.
– Your joint is impossible to move.
– Fever, or you are feeling flushed, hot and sweaty (your temperature is over 38°C or 100.4°F).

 **Call NHS Direct**

**No**

*See the opposite page*

**NHS Direct** CALL 24 HOURS ON **0845 4647**

Is this the first time you have felt this pain in your joints?

 Yes **Call NHS Direct**

 **No**

Are other joints hot, swollen and painful as well?

 Yes **Call NHS Direct**

 **No**

Does the pain start after the same repeated movements like typing, using a screwdriver or playing tennis?

 Yes **Self-care**

You may have a repetitive strain injury which will respond to rest or alternative forms of exercise. Anti-inflammatory medicines do help. **Ask your pharmacist** for advice.

 **No**

Does the pain gradually get worse as the day goes on?

 Yes **Self-care**

You may have osteoarthritis which is caused by wear and tear. **Ask your pharmacist** for advice.

 **No**

**Self-care advice**

- It is important to rest the affected area.
- Complete rest may make the condition worse.
- Regular painkillers, such as paracetamol or ibuprofen, may help.
- A cold compress will help reduce swelling.
- An ice pack or bag of frozen peas wrapped in a tea towel can be applied to the area for no longer than 5 minutes. Repeat every hour.
- If the pain continues or new symptoms develop, call **NHS Direct**.
- If you are still worried, call **NHS Direct**.

**Before ringing NHS Direct or 999, it would be helpful if you think about the following and are ready to answer the questions if asked.**
- How long you or the person you are calling about have been unwell.
- Your or their temperature (if possible).
- Any medicines you or they are taking at the moment.
- Any illnesses, such as rheumatoid arthritis, you or they have had before.

*Joint pains*

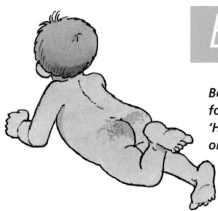

# Baby rashes

*Before going through the following questions, check 'How do I know if my baby is ill?' on page 5.*

**Is the rash:**
- dark red?
- mainly on the elbows, legs and buttocks?

**Does it change its appearance and place on the skin?**

 **Yes**

### Call NHS Direct

Serious problems are rare but these irregularly-shaped dark-red spots could follow an allergic reaction to infection or some disorder of the blood. Call **NHS Direct**.

Go to *Purpura* on page 109 for more information.

 **No**

**Does the child have a fever, are they flushed, hot and sweaty (is their temperature over 38°C or 100.4°F)?**

 **Yes**

Go to *Rashes with fever* on page 88 for more information.

 **No**

**Is the rash a crusty wax scale on the scalp?**

 **Yes**

### Self-care

Cradle cap is a form of eczema. It responds well to simply rubbing the affected parts of the scalp with olive oil. Leave it on overnight before washing it off with a mild shampoo in the morning. **See your pharmacist**.

Go to *Cradle cap* on page 94 for more information.

**No**

**Is the rash mainly in the nappy area?**

 **Yes**

### Self-care

Rashes in the nappy area are common but can be eased or avoided completely.
- As far as possible change each nappy after it has become dirty.
- As much as possible, leave the nappy off, particularly any plastic pants. Dry, cool skin rarely gets nappy rash.
- An angry red rash which won't respond or spreads beyond the nappy area may be a fungal infection (Candida).

**Ask your pharmacist or health visitor**.

Go to *Nappy rash* on page 108 for more information.

**No**

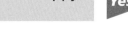
*See the opposite page*

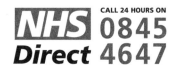 **CALL 24 HOURS ON** 0845 4647

82

Is the rash red, itchy, flaky and in more than one place?

 **Yes**

**Self-care**

Eczema covers a range of skin problems. There is a wide range of products which will help stop the itchiness and keep the skin moist. Follow your doctor's advice on how to use topical steroid creams.

Call **NHS Direct**, but call your **doctor** if:
– the eczema is spreading very quickly;
– the skin is becoming infected; or
– there is severe pain.

Go to *Eczema* on page 95 for more information.

 **No**

Is the rash blotchy, red and difficult to feel?

**Yes**

**Self-care**

All babies and children will have a heat rash at some time. No treatment is needed other than lowering their temperature by moving them away from the heat, removing their clothes and keeping them in a cool room.

Go to *Heat rash* on page 97 for more information.

 **No**

**Self-care advice**

- A rash alone is unlikely to be serious.
- Encourage the child to rest and watch them closely for signs of illness.
- Make sure the child is drinking plenty of fluids.
- Paracetamol (for example, Calpol) may be helpful if the child is restless.
- **Ask your pharmacist** to recommend a cream that may provide some relief.
- Calamine lotion may give relief for a short time.
- Two tablespoons of bicarbonate of soda added to bath water may relieve any itching.
- If the condition gets worse or if any other symptoms develop, call **NHS Direct**.

**Before ringing NHS Direct or 999, it would be helpful if you think about the following and are ready to answer the questions if asked.**
- Their symptoms (the questions you answered 'Yes' to).
- Their temperature (if possible).
- When they last had anything to eat or drink.
- Any medicines they are taking at the moment.
- Any allergies you know of.
- Any serious illnesses they have had before.

www.nhsdirect.nhs.uk

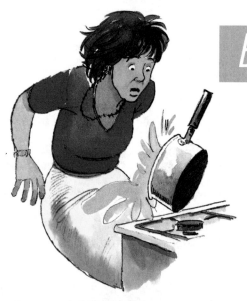

# Burns and scalds

*This advice is suitable for adults and children.*

| | | |
|---|---|---|
| Is there any shortness of breath? |  Yes ▶ | **Dial 999**  |

Inhaling fumes or flames can damage the airways. If they are short of breath, **dial 999**.

 No ▼

| | | |
|---|---|---|
| Are there any other injuries such as electric shock or broken bones? |  Yes ▶ | **Dial 999**  |

If the burn came from an electric shock or there are broken bones from a fall, **dial 999**.

 No ▼

| | | |
|---|---|---|
| Is the burn or scald area larger than the size of the adult's or child's own hand? |  Yes ▶ | **Call NHS Direct**  |

It is easy to underestimate the area of a burn or scald. If it is larger than the size of the person's hand, call **NHS Direct**.

 No ▼

| | | |
|---|---|---|
| Is the burn or scald on the face or around the mouth? |  Yes ▶ | **Call NHS Direct**  |

Burns or scalds around the mouth may mean that they have inhaled the fumes or flames. Call **NHS Direct**.

▼

*See the opposite page*

**NHS Direct** CALL 24 HOURS ON **0845 4647**

Do you feel you need more advice on how to treat this burn? **Yes** ▶ **Call NHS Direct**

**No** ▼

## Self-care advice

- Take off any bracelets, rings, shoes, necklaces or watches which may restrict blood flow.
- Cool the affected area with running water for 15 minutes.
- Do not apply any creams or ointments.
- Cover with clingfilm, if available, or a clean, dry, non-fluffy cotton cloth (for example, a handkerchief).
- Take some painkillers, such as paracetamol.
- If the condition gets worse or new symptoms develop, call **NHS Direct**.
- If you are still worried, call **NHS Direct**.

Before ringing **NHS Direct** or **999**, it would be helpful if you think about the following and are ready to answer the questions if asked.
- When the burn or scald happened.
- If it involved an electric shock.
- If they are unconscious.
- If there are any broken bones.
- The approximate size of the burn or scald.

*Burns and scalds*

www.nhsdirect.nhs.uk

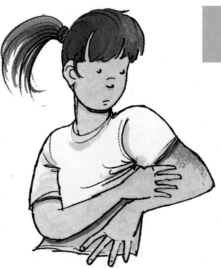

# Itchy rashes

**Is the rash red, smooth, or slightly raised (can you feel it)?**  **Yes**

**No**

---

## Self-care

Hives can be a reaction to food (for example, shellfish and strawberries), medicines, plants (for example, nettles) or a viral infection. The rash will usually disappear in a few hours without any treatment. Call **NHS Direct** if the rash has not disappeared after 24 hours. **Dial 999** if they have any breathing difficulties or they cannot swallow.

Go to *Hives, urticaria and nettle rash* on page 98 for more information.

---

**Is the rash only at the lips and mouth corners?**  **Yes**

**No**

*See the opposite page*

---

## Self-care

It could be a cold sore.
- Once infected, avoid sudden changes in temperature and sun exposure.
- Use simple painkillers such as paracetamol (for example, Calpol, but not aspirin in children under 16 years).
- Use a lip salve before going into bright sunlight.
- Acyclovir cream (for example, Zovirax) **from your pharmacist** will limit the outbreak.

Go to *Cold sores* on page 93 for more information.

---

**NHS Direct**
CALL 24 HOURS ON
**0845 4647**

Is the rash shaped like a ring and is it flaky?  **Yes**

### Self-care

Ringworm (tinea) can affect many parts of the body, particularly the groin and scalp. Keep the area well ventilated and dry. Use an antifungal cream or shampoo which you can get **from your pharmacist**, and keep your face cloth and towel separate. Ringworm is infectious.

Go to *Ringworm* on page 110 for more information.

**No**

Is the rash itchy and on the fingers, hand or wrist?  **Yes**

### Self-care

Scabies is caused by a mite which burrows just under the skin, often between the fingers, wrists, elbows and the genital areas. You can get ointments **from your pharmacist**. The body from the neck down will need to be covered with the ointment for 24 hours and all clothing and bedding should be washed thoroughly.

Go to *Scabies* on page 110 for more information.

**No**

Is it raised with one or more raised patches in the same area?  **Yes**

### Self-care

At first, insect bites can be mistaken for more serious things. If you look very closely, you can generally see the small hole of the actual bite. **See your pharmacist**.

Go to *Insect bites* on page 100 for more information.

**No**

### Self-care advice

- A rash alone is unlikely to be serious.
- Encourage the person to rest and watch closely for signs of illness.
- Make sure the person is drinking plenty of fluids.
- Paracetamol (for example, Calpol for children) may be helpful if they are restless.
- **Ask your pharmacist** to recommend a cream that may provide some relief.
- Calamine lotion may give relief for a short time.
- Two tablespoons of bicarbonate of soda added to bath water may relieve any itching.
- If the condition gets worse or if any other symptoms develop, call **NHS Direct**.
- If you are still worried, call **NHS Direct**.

**Before ringing NHS Direct or 999, it would be helpful if you think about the following and are ready to answer the questions if asked.**
- Your symptoms (the questions you answered 'Yes' to), or the symptoms of the person you are calling about.
- Your or their temperature (if possible).
- When you or they last had anything to eat or drink.
- Any medicines you or they are taking at the moment.
- Any allergies you know of.
- Any serious illnesses you or they have had before.

www.nhsdirect.nhs.uk

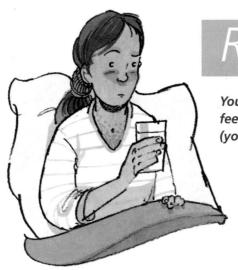

# Rashes with fever

*You may have a **fever** if you are feeling flushed, hot and sweaty (your temperature is over 38°C or 100.4°F).*

Is the person developing a rash that does not fade when you press a glass tumbler or finger against it?

 **Yes**

**Dial 999**

 **No**

Are the spots red and difficult to feel and is there a cough or runny nose?

 **Yes**

## Self-care

This is probably a viral rash.
Rashes in children are common.
- Keep the child cool.
- Use paracetamol (for example, Calpol) for fever and aches and pains.
- Cough medicines may ease ticklish throats. Place a bowl of water in the room to increase the humidity.
- Avoid dehydration. Feverish small children rapidly lose water. It also makes a ticklish cough worse.
  If the person has not been vaccinated with the MMR vaccination, a viral rash like this could be measles.

Go to *Measles* on page 103 for more information.

**No**

Are there swellings on the neck?

 **Yes**

## Self-care

This may be a viral infection which can be treated at home. If the person has not been vaccinated with the MMR vaccination, a viral rash like this could be German measles (rubella).

Go to *German measles (rubella)* on page 96 for more information.

**No**

*See the opposite page*

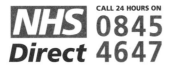
**NHS Direct** CALL 24 HOURS ON **0845 4647**

**If you can feel the spots, are they turning into small blisters?**

**No**

## Self-care

It could be chickenpox. Intensely itchy, tiny clear blisters soon follow. Fresh red spots are usually seen next to blisters and crusts.

- Most children are free from chickenpox in less than two weeks.
- Dab calamine lotion on the infected spots which should ease the itching.
- Use cool baths without soap every three to four hours for the first couple of days. Add a few tablespoons of bicarbonate of soda to the bath water.
- Antihistamines are available **from your pharmacist**. These help reduce itching and promote sleep, so use them just before bed time.
- Paracetamol (for example, Calpol) helps reduce the fever.
- Ice lollies help lower temperature and provide sugar and water while reducing the irritation of a mouth infection. They can be used for children over four years old.
- If you are pregnant or think you could be, call **NHS Direct**.

Go to *Chickenpox* on page 93 for more information.

## Self-care advice

- A rash alone is unlikely to be serious.
- Encourage the person to rest and watch them closely for signs of illness.
- Make sure the person is drinking plenty of fluids.
- Paracetamol (for example, Calpol for children) may be helpful if they are restless.
- **Ask your pharmacist** to recommend a cream that may provide some relief.
- Calamine lotion will give relief for a short time.
- Two tablespoons of bicarbonate of soda added to bath water may relieve any itching.
- If the condition gets worse or if any other symptoms develop, call **NHS Direct**.
- If you are still worried, call **NHS Direct**.

**Before ringing NHS Direct or 999, it would be helpful if you think about the following and are ready to answer the questions if asked.**

- Your symptoms (the questions you answered 'Yes' to), or the symptoms of the person you are calling about.
- Your or their temperature (if possible).
- When you or they last had anything to eat or drink.
- Any medicines you or they are taking at the moment.
- Any allergies you know of.
- Any serious illnesses you or they have had before.

*Rashes with fever*

www.nhsdirect.nhs.uk

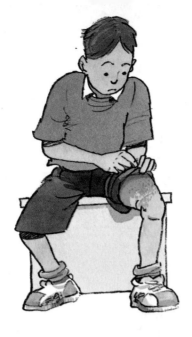

# Rashes

*This advice is suitable
for adults and children.*

Do you or they have a fever, are you or they feeling flushed, hot and sweaty (is the temperature over 38°C or 100.4°F)?  **Yes** → Go to *Rashes with fever* on page 88 for more information.

 **No**

Do you or they have a rash which is red or purple and does not fade when you press a glass tumbler or a finger against it?  **Yes** → **Dial 999**

 **No**

Do you or they have either of the following symptoms?
– Light hurts the eyes.
– It is difficult to bend the neck.  **Yes** → **Call NHS Direct**

 **No**

Does the rash come and go and is it:
– dark red?
– mainly on the elbows, legs and buttocks?  **Yes** → **Call NHS Direct**

Serious problems are rare but these irregularly-shaped dark-red spots could follow an allergic reaction to infection or some disorder of the blood. Call **NHS Direct**.

Go to *Purpura* on page 109 for more information.

 **No**

*See the opposite page*

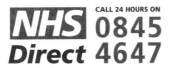 **CALL 24 HOURS ON 0845 4647**

Is it red and crusty, or are there weeping sores on the face?

**Yes**

**No**

### Call NHS Direct

It may be impetigo which is more common in children but is also seen in adults.
It is infectious.
Use separate washing materials and ease any pain with paracetamol (for example, Calpol for children) (not aspirin in any child under 16 years). If the rash will not go away, your doctor can give you a treatment for the infection.

### Go to *Impetigo* on page 99 for more information.

---

Is the person a baby (under one year old)?

**Yes**

**No**

### Self-care

Most rashes in children are harmless and can be treated at home with **advice from your pharmacist**. Keep an open mind for more serious illnesses and phone **NHS Direct** if you are not sure after reading the rest of the information.

### Go to *Baby rashes* on page 82 for more information.

---

Is the rash itchy?

**Yes**

**No**

Most itchy rashes are relatively harmless but are sometimes infectious.

### Go to *Itchy rashes* on page 86 for more information.

---

### Self-care advice ➕

- A rash alone is unlikely to be serious.
- Encourage the person to rest and watch closely for signs of illness.
- Make sure the person is drinking plenty of fluids.
- Paracetamol (for example, Calpol for children) may be helpful if the person is restless.
- **Ask your pharmacist** to recommend a cream that may provide some relief.
- Calamine lotion may give relief for a short time.
- Some people may find it helpful to add two tablespoons of bicarbonate of soda to bath water as it may relieve any itching.
- If the condition gets worse or if any other symptoms develop, call **NHS Direct**.
- If you are still worried, call **NHS Direct**.

**Before ringing NHS Direct or 999, it would be helpful if you think about the following and are ready to answer the questions if asked.**

- Your symptoms (the questions you answered 'Yes' to), or the symptoms of the person you are calling about.
- Your or their temperature (if possible).
- When you or they last had anything to eat or drink.
- Any medicines you or they are taking at the moment.
- Any allergies you know of.
- Any serious illnesses you or they have had before.

# Glossary of conditions

## *Breast cancer*

*Breast cancer is the most common form of cancer in women, causing over 14,000 deaths each year in the UK.*

### Symptoms

■ You should report any changes in your breasts, such as lumps, pain, hardness, leaking from the nipple or a dragging feeling, to your doctor. You should also report puckering of the skin, a rash around the nipple, one breast getting larger or lower than the other, or lumps under the armpit.

**Causes**  We don't know exactly why breast cancer happens but there are certain women at higher risk than others.

– Those with a mother or sister or other close relative who has breast cancer.

– Older women – breast cancer is rare under the age of 40.

– Women whose periods started early and have had a late (after the age of 55) menopause (sometimes known as 'the change').

– Never having been pregnant, or having your first baby after the age of 30, are also risk factors.

– Overweight menopausal women.

– Women in 'Western' countries.

– The oral contraceptive pill does not increase a woman's risk of developing breast cancer.

**Prevention**  There is no real protection except early detection. Check your breasts each month so that you can recognise changes if they happen – 'be breast aware'. Lying on the bed is a good place to check. Use the flat of your palm to check and compare each breast. Use a mirror to see if they look any different. Ask your partner if they have noticed any difference. Remember that 90% of lumps are harmless but early diagnosis of breast cancer can make all the difference.

Mammography (a special X-ray) is available on the NHS to all women between the ages of 50 and 64 years. At the moment it is available every three years. Your GP will be able to arrange this if necessary. Even so, a small number of breast cancers will not show up on X-ray, so you still need to keep checking.

### Self-care

■ Keeping healthy is important even with breast cancer. Early diagnosis improves the chances of survival.

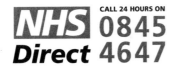

**NHS Direct**  CALL 24 HOURS ON **0845 4647**

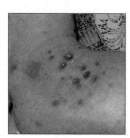

## Chickenpox

*Children exposed to the virus develop chickenpox seven to 21 days later. In most cases there are no symptoms before the rash appears.*

### Symptoms

- A mild fever, stomach ache and feeling run-down can occur a day or two before the flat, red rash appears. This generally begins on the scalp, face and back but can spread to anywhere, although it is rarely seen on the palms of the hands or soles of the feet.
- Intensely itchy, tiny clear blisters soon follow.
- Fresh red spots are usually seen next to blisters and crusts.
- Most children are free from chickenpox in less than two weeks.

**Causes** This virus spreads quickly, especially between children. Sneezing, coughing, contaminated clothing and direct contact with the open blisters are all ways of catching this relatively harmless infection.

**Prevention** There is no licensed vaccine in this country at the moment.

**Complications** Complications are very rare, although chickenpox can occasionally lead to encephalitis (inflammation of the brain), meningitis or pneumonia.

Serious complications are more common in children who are taking medicines, such as steroids, as they can lower the body's immune defence system. Speak to your doctor's surgery for advice now.

### Self-care

- Use cool baths without soap every three to four hours for the first couple of days. Adding a few tablespoons of bicarbonate of soda to the bath water may help.
- Ask your pharmacist for something to provide temporary relief.
- Cotton socks on children's hands will prevent too much scratching, which can lead to infection.
- Paracetamol (for example, Calpol) helps reduce the fever. Do not give aspirin to children under 16.
- Ice lollies help lower temperature, provide sugar and water and, at the same time, reduce the irritation of a mouth infection. They may be used for children over four.

**More information** A child will be infectious until the last spot has crusted over.

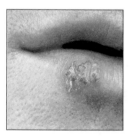

## Cold sores (herpes)

*Herpes is a virus which lives in nerve endings within the skin. It normally appears felt around the corners of the mouth, with crusty, oozing blisters.*

### Symptoms

- A tingling, itchy feeling is usually felt just before the rash forms.
- Tiny blisters appear, usually at the lips where they join the skin.
- The blisters become sore and itchy.

### Cold sores (herpes) continued

■ They then crust over and last about one week before disappearing.

■ They can return at any time.

**Causes**  Kissing or other contact with someone infected with herpes. The virus is infectious, particularly when the blister is erupting.

**Prevention**  There is not much you can do to prevent catching a cold sore other than avoid kissing people who have obvious signs of it on their face. Once infected, avoid sudden changes in temperature or going out into the sun.

**Complications**  There is a related form of herpes which can infect the genitals and which can be transmitted through oral sex.

### Self-care

■ Use simple painkillers such as paracetamol.

■ Use a lip salve with a high sun protection factor (SPF) before going into bright sunlight.

■ Acyclovir cream (for example, Zovirax) will limit the outbreak if you start using it as early as possible. Ask your pharmacist for advice.

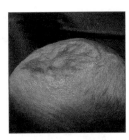
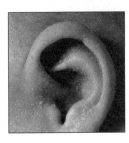

## Cradle cap

*A harmless white and yellow waxy scale which builds up on the scalp.*

### Symptoms

■ A thick white and yellow waxy scale builds up on the scalp. There is no bleeding or obvious irritation unless you have been too rough in trying to remove it. There is no fever and the child is perfectly well.

**Causes**  Like many other forms of eczema, the cause is unknown.

**Prevention**  Regular cleaning will prevent it in most cases.

**Complications**  There are no serious complications.

### Self-care

■ A form of eczema, it responds well to simply rubbing the affected parts of the scalp with olive oil. Leave it on overnight before washing it off with a mild shampoo in the morning.

■ You can get shampoos from your pharmacist but you should try rubbing with olive oil first. Ask your pharmacist for advice.

## Cystitis

*Women suffer most from this infection of the bladder, which makes you pass water more often and may sting when you do. Men appear to get off lightly because of the greater distance between the anus, where most of the bacteria come from, and the urethra, through which urine is passed.*

### Symptoms

■ A stinging sensation when passing water.

■ A feeling of needing to pass water very often.

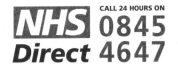
CALL 24 HOURS ON
**NHS Direct** 0845 4647

**Causes** The most common cause is a bacterial infection from the anus. You may also get it if you have kidney stones or diabetes.

**Prevention** Drinking plenty of fluids helps to prevent cystitis in the first place.

### Self-care

■ Drink slightly acidic drinks such as cranberry juice, lemon squash or pure orange juice.

■ Try a mixture of potassium citrate, which you can get from your pharmacist.

■ Sex can cause cystitis in women. Urinating after sex can help to flush out any bacteria that may have entered the urethra.

### Note

Call **NHS Direct** if:

– you still feel infected after one day;

– there is any blood in your urine; or

– you are pregnant.

Take a urine sample from your first visit to the toilet in the morning to your GP surgery. Use a clean, well-rinsed bottle.

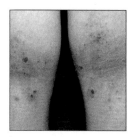

## *Eczema*

*Basically, it is inflammation of the skin which produces dry, flaky skin, more often on the inside of joints such as the elbow. It is more common in young people and old people. The term 'dermatitis' is exactly the same thing but tends to be used when the eczema is caused by contact with a chemical or other substances.*

### Symptoms

■ Atopic eczema is an allergic condition. People who suffer from other allergies, such as hay fever, are also prone to eczema. It can affect any part of the body, but the inside of the elbows, knees and wrists are the most common sites.

■ The dry, flaky skin can come and go but tends to be worse in winter or during cold weather.

■ Contact dermatitis can be very severe, with the skin becoming deeply inflamed, leading to skin loss. The underlying deep skin looks red and angry. Infection is often the next step.

■ Seborrhoeic dermatitis is the name for eczema that affects the scalp and eyebrows. A thick, yellow, greasy scale builds up, leading to heavy dandruff.

**Causes** Atopic eczema is probably an inherited condition. The inflammation flares up as a response to some allergy although it may never be identified. Hair dye, watches made of nickel, jewellery and washing powders are all known to cause contact dermatitis in people who are prone to infection. Seborrhoeic dermatitis may be a fungal infection, although it could also be an extreme form of allergy that affects the hairy parts of the body.

### Eczema continued

**Prevention**  It makes sense to identify and avoid those substances, materials or chemicals which trigger the eczema.

Keep the skin moist with emollient ointments (soothing ointments). Your pharmacist will advise you.

Use a bath-water additive which contains moisturising oils.

**Complications**  Skin may become infected, particularly in very young children. Unfortunately, topical steroid creams, which can be effective in treating eczema, also make the skin more prone to infection. Contact dermatitis can be so severe that the skin is lost in the affected area, leading to infection and scarring. Not surprisingly this can be intensely itchy and painful. Using steroids too often or in too high doses can be dangerous. Always follow the suggested dose on the pack and ask your pharmacist for advice.

### Self-care

■ There is a wide range of products which will help stop the itchiness and keep the skin moist.

■ Topical steroid creams may be helpful. If the eczema is mild, ask your pharmacist for advice. If it is severe, get advice from your GP.

■ Scratching and itchiness can be reduced by keeping the skin moist and taking antihistamine tablets or medicine. This is useful for young children as it also has a mild sedative effect, helping them to sleep better.

### Note: Action – *Call* NHS Direct *but speak to your doctor if:*

– the eczema is spreading very quickly;

– the skin is becoming infected; or

– there is severe pain.

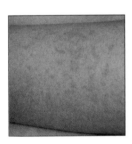

# German measles (rubella)

*This is now uncommon thanks to the Measles, Mumps and Rubella (MMR) vaccine.*

### Symptoms

■ The person is rarely ill but will have a slightly raised temperature and swollen glands on the neck and base of the skull.

■ The pinhead-sized, flat red spots last about two days and need no treatment. Paracetamol will help reduce the slight fever.

**Causes**  The virus is very contagious and will spread quickly in people who are not immune.

**Prevention**  Vaccination for girls and boys is safe and effective.

**Complications**  Very rarely the virus that causes German measles (rubella) will cause an inflammation of the brain (encephalitis). The real danger may come in later life if an unvaccinated woman becomes infected with German measles (rubella) while pregnant as it can affect the development of the baby. For this reason alone, both boys and girls should be immunised with this very safe vaccine.

### Self-care

■ Paracetamol will reduce the mild fever.

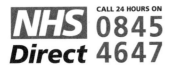
**NHS Direct**  CALL 24 HOURS ON **0845 4647**

## Hangovers

*A hangover can be so bad you actually think there is something seriously wrong with you, especially if it is the first time it has ever happened.*

### Symptoms

■ Headache, nausea, tiredness and thirst are the most common symptoms.

**Causes**  Dehydration is the main cause. Alcohol acts as a 'diuretic' which causes the kidneys to lose water. Some alcoholic drinks contain toxins which act as mild poisons. Too much red wine tends to cause headaches for this reason. The quality of sleep while you are drunk is always poor as the alcohol interferes with the normal sleep pattern. This will make you feel as though you have not slept the next morning.

**Prevention**  The best way to avoid a hangover is not to drink too much. Drinking a few glasses of water before you go to sleep will also help. Switch to low-alcohol or non-alcoholic drinks towards the end of the evening.

**Complications**  Hangovers are rarely dangerous, but regularly drinking alcohol again when you wake up to ease the symptoms can lead to alcohol abuse. People underestimate just how long alcohol stays in the bloodstream after a night's drinking and may well be still over the legal limit for driving the next day.

### Self-care

■ Drink plenty of water, take paracetamol and, if possible, have a nap later on to make up for the poor quality of sleep.

**Note**  If you regularly suffer from hangovers, it is highly likely that you are abusing alcohol and may be becoming dependent on it. If people are commenting on your drinking, you are becoming defensive over it, your work or home relationships are suffering or you are drinking early in the day, you should get advice from **NHS Direct** or contact a support group such as Alcoholics Anonymous.

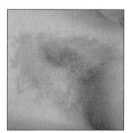

## Heat rash

*All babies and children will have a rash at some time (sometimes called 'heat rash').*

### Symptoms

■ It looks like a fine pattern of tiny red spots which come and go but tend to disappear if their temperature is lowered.

■ The baby will be perfectly well.

**Causes**  A cold or a viral infection are the most common causes. Too many clothes or bedding will also cause it.

**Complications**  If your baby gets too hot, cool them down immediately by removing their clothes and keep them in a cool room.

### Self-care

■ No treatment is needed, other than lowering their temperature with paracetamol syrup (for example, Calpol).

## Hiatus hernia and heartburn

*This is the reflux (bringing up) of stomach acid into the gullet. The condition used to be more than just a nuisance before the appearance of modern drugs, which reduce the production of stomach acid.*

### Symptoms

■ A burning sensation (heartburn) behind the breastbone which is made worse by bending over or lying flat. There may also be an acid taste that is brought up from the stomach. There can be difficulty in swallowing, with repeated reflux of stomach acid.

**Causes** The neck of the stomach rolls into the chest, allowing stomach acid to pass into the gullet.

**Prevention** You can't prevent a hiatus hernia but you can ease the symptoms. You can prevent many of the symptoms by:

– controlling your weight;

– controlling how much you eat; and

– not smoking.

**Complications** Constant acid irritation of the gullet can make swallowing difficult.

### Self-care

■ Avoid foods that trigger attacks, such as rich and fatty foods. Take indigestion remedies (antacids) and drink milk to relieve the symptoms. Sleep with an extra pillow to stop the acid reflux.

## Hives, urticaria and nettle rash

### Symptoms

■ Hives are small, often itchy, **raised** red spots which you can feel and are rarely serious, unless you also have any breathing problems.

■ The rash will usually disappear in a few hours without any treatment.

**Causes** It is most often caused by certain foods and plants (for example, nettles) but may be caused by a viral infection.

**Complications** Rarely the rash is severe and associated with breathing difficulties. This is an emergency. Dial 999.

### Self-care

■ A pharmacist may be able to recommend a cream or medicine that could provide some relief.

■ If there is any shortness of breath, dial 999.

**NHS Direct** CALL 24 HOURS ON 0845 4647

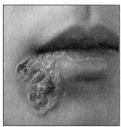

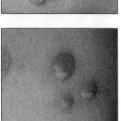

## Impetigo

*Bacterial infections of the skin are fairly common. Impetigo is more common in children but is also seen in adults. It is infectious but is no longer a serious threat, thanks to antibiotics.*

### Symptoms

■ It usually starts as a small red spot which gradually increases in size.

■ The top becomes crusty and weeps.

■ It is often found around the corners of the mouth and face, but can also be found on the rest of the body.

**Causes**  It is infectious and is caught from direct contact with infected children or adults. It is also spread through sharing face cloths and towels.

**Prevention**  Use separate washing materials.

**Complications**  It spreads much more quickly in people who are generally run-down with illness or stress.

### Self-care

■ Clean the spots with a damp tissue. Give painkillers, such as paracetamol, for any pain.

■ If the spots will not go away, you may need antibiotics. Contact your GP during regular surgery hours.

## Indigestion

*Indigestion is more common in middle-aged people, after eating heavy meals or drinking alcohol, and is often worse at night. Regurgitation or reflux is painful although rarely dangerous. Stomach acid escapes into the gullet, causing chest pain. It can be mistaken for a heart attack. Severe reflux can happen with a hiatus hernia (see page 98).*

### Symptoms

■ A vague pain below the ribcage, extending into the throat.

■ An acid taste in the mouth.

■ Too much wind.

### Causes

– Eating a heavy meal or drinking alcohol.

– 'Rich' food that often contains a lot of fat.

– Smoking too much.

– A leaking valve at the neck of the stomach (hiatus hernia).

### Prevention

– Avoid food which you know can bring on an attack.

– Sleep with your upper body propped up with pillows.

– Avoid eating just before bedtime.

www.nhsdirect.nhs.uk

### Indigestion continued

– Eat small meals more often.

– Avoid aspirin and drugs like ibuprofen (non-steroidal anti-inflammatory drugs).

**Complications** Most indigestion is harmless but annoying. The acid refluxing into the throat does not appear to cause any serious damage. The greatest danger is ignoring repeated attacks or confusing them with a heart attack. Get medical advice if your symptoms won't go away or if they get worse.

### Self-care

■ Your pharmacist will advise about indigestion remedies (antacids and other medicines).

■ Avoid taking large amounts of sodium bicarbonate (bicarbonate of soda) as this is turned into salt in the body.

■ A glass of milk before bed can help.

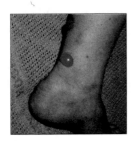

## Insect bites and stings

*At first, insect bites can be mistaken for more serious things.*

### Symptoms

■ If you look very closely, you can generally see the small hole of the actual bite. The rash or individual 'spot' is usually itchy and may swell, particularly if it is a bite from a horsefly (cleg).

**Causes** 'Midges', horseflies, bees, wasps, centipedes, ants, lice and so on. The list is long but thankfully there are no killers within the UK.

**Prevention** Insect repellents work. If you think you have lice, ask your pharmacist for advice (see *Lice* on page 102).

**Complications** Some people are strongly allergic to bites and stings and can be very ill. If there is any shortness of breath, dial 999. Bites can become infected by scratching.

### Self-care

■ Although bites are itchy and sometimes painful, they are rarely dangerous and need only some antihistamine or local anaesthetic cream from your pharmacist. Ask your pharmacist for advice.

■ The redness and swelling are usually due to the allergy rather than an infection. Antibiotics are rarely needed in the first 48 hours.

■ Call your doctor if the symptoms will not go away.

## Irritable bowel syndrome (IBS)

*Diagnosis is based on ruling out other conditions. There is no accurate test for IBS. It affects three times as many women as men. Symptoms can start at any age but are more common between the ages of 15 and 40. Stress and lifestyle are major factors. The cause remains unknown. It is rarely, if ever, fatal.*

**NHS Direct** CALL 24 HOURS ON **0845 4647**

## Symptoms

Along with a lot of wind, the symptoms of IBS are:

- constipation that comes and goes;
- diarrhoea; and
- a colicky tummy (abdominal) pain.

**Causes** The cause is unknown but it may be stress-related.

## Prevention

- Go for a high-fibre diet containing whole-grain bread, rice and pasta.
- Eating plenty of fresh fruit can produce a remarkable long-term improvement in symptoms.
- Dairy products are often the bad guys. Try cutting out cheese, milk, chocolate, butter and cream from your diet for a few weeks to see if there is any improvement.
- Red meat, not just beef, can often seriously upset your bowel if you are prone to IBS.
- Use herbs that are known to ease the symptoms of IBS, for example, peppermint.
- Stress can be a big factor.
- Exercise is valuable. It increases bowel activity which reduces bloating and swelling.
- Nicotine also makes IBS much worse so you should try to cut down or stop smoking altogether.
- Small amounts of alcohol can actually help to improve your bowel movements.
- Tea contains as much caffeine as coffee. Both can cause diarrhoea in people who are prone to IBS. Coffee also contains an unknown substance that causes bowel cramps.

## Self-care

- Drugs are the last resort and only have a temporary effect. Codeine relieves the spasm but can cause constipation. Peppermint oil is the basic ingredient of many drugs prescribed by your GP for IBS. Antidiarrhoeal drugs and laxatives can help but you should not use them for a long time.
- The pain and discomfort of IBS can sometimes be relieved by a hot-water bottle which fits snuggly against your stomach.

### However, see your doctor if:

- the home treatment doesn't work after two weeks;
- you pass blood in your motions;
- your bowel motions are very dark or black or are covered with mucus; or
- there is an unexplained weight loss.

## More information

For more information contact:
British Digestive Foundation
3 St Andrews Place
London NW1 4LB.

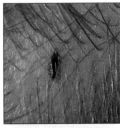
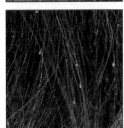

## Lice

*Head lice are small six-legged, wingless insects, pinhead size when they hatch, less than match-head size when fully grown, and grey or brown in colour. Female lice lay eggs in sacs which hatch in seven to 10 days.*

*Lice are the insects that can be seen moving on, or close to, the scalp. Nits are the pearly-white empty egg shells of head lice that are left stuck to hair shafts after the insects have hatched. Nits may still be found even after all the lice have been cleared, but you should not start treatment unless you find living, moving lice.*

### Symptoms

■ Lice are nearly always completely harmless. They do not always cause itching, particularly when they have just arrived on the head.

**Causes** Social status means nothing to lice. They are common among children and infection has nothing to do with dirty hair. Head lice cannot fly, jump or swim but are spread by clambering from head to head. Anyone with hair can catch them.

### Detection

– Head lice are well camouflaged and hide when they are disturbed by combing. If there aren't many of them, it can be difficult to find them.
– To check for lice, comb wet hair regularly with a fine-tooth comb. Use a conditioner to make combing easier.

**Self-care** Do not use any form of treatment unless you find a living, moving louse. There are two treatment options.

■ **Lotions using insecticides** Check all close family and friends by the 'wet combing' method and treat anyone who is found to have lice at the same time, to prevent re-infection. Make sure you have enough lotion to treat all those affected and follow the instructions on the packet carefully.

■ **The 'Bug Busting' treatment method** This aims at removing live lice by combing through the hair and physically removing any lice you find. To be successful, you must be thorough and patient – as described in the 'Bug Busting' kit you can get from some pharmacies, and by mail order from Community Hygiene Concern (Helpline: 020 8341 7167).

A recent study suggested that insecticide lotion was much more effective than 'Bug Busting'.

### More information

You can get a leaflet, *The Prevention and Treatment of Head Lice*, from:
Department of Health
PO Box 777
London SE1 6XH.
Or you can e-mail them at doh@prologistics.co.uk

**NHS Direct** CALL 24 HOURS ON 0845 4647

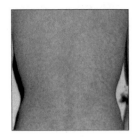

# *Measles*

*Children are most vulnerable to this highly contagious viral infection. This is now very rare in the UK, due to the MMR vaccination.*

### Symptoms

Symptoms usually develop in a well-established order.

- A mild to severe temperature of around 39°C or 102.2°F.
- Tiredness and general fatigue.
- A poor appetite.
- A runny nose and sneezing.
- An irritable dry cough.
- Red eyes and sensitivity to light.
- Tiny white spots in the mouth and throat.
- A blotchy red rash that starts behind the ears, spreads to the face and then to the rest of the body and lasts for up to seven days.

**Causes**  It takes around 10 to 12 days for the virus to make its presence felt after infection from another child. Physical contact, sneezing and clothing contaminated with nasal secretions (mucus from the nose) all help to spread this infection.

**Prevention**  Although immunisation rates are now very high, you should isolate your child from other children if you think they may be infected. Immunised children and those who have already caught measles are virtually immune.

**Complications**  Meningitis and pneumonia are rare but serious complications. More commonly, eyes and ears develop secondary infections which may need antibiotics from your doctor.

### Self-care

- Once the rash starts it is a matter of treating the symptoms.
- Check the child's temperature.
- Use paracetamol syrup (for example, Calpol) for fever and aches and pains.
- Light sensitivity can be helped by reducing sunlight or electric lights in the room.
- Use a ball of damp cotton wool to clean away any crustiness around the eyes.
- Cough medicines are of little value but do ease ticklish throats. Try placing a bowl of water in the room.
- Avoid dehydration. Feverish small children rapidly lose water. It also makes a cough worse.
- Some people may find it helpful to try one teaspoon of lemon juice and two teaspoons of honey in a glass of warm water.
- Ideally, you should keep your child away from others for at least seven days after the start of the rash.
- After four days the child usually feels better.

**More information**  To protect your child against measles, make sure that they are vaccinated with the MMR vaccination.

www.nhsdirect.nhs.uk

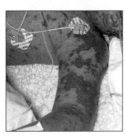

*Later stage of the rash as it appears on a dark skin.*

# Meningitis and septicaemia

*These are rare illnesses which cause inflammation of the brain lining, which can be fatal. Unfortunately, the symptoms can be easily mistaken for flu or a bad cold. Worse still, it is more difficult to be certain with babies and young children. If you are not sure, you must call* **NHS Direct**. *The Hib and meningitis C immunisation has reduced the number of people suffering from some types of meningitis and septicaemia. Unfortunately, we do not have vaccines for every type of meningitis and septicaemia, so we all still need to watch out for the symptoms.*

## Symptoms

Babies under two.

■ They can be difficult to wake.

■ Their cry may be high-pitched and different from normal.

■ They may vomit repeatedly, not just after feeds.

■ They may refuse feeds, either from the bottle, from the breast or by spoon.

■ Their skin may appear pale or blotchy, possibly with a red or purple rash which does not fade when you press a glass tumbler or a finger against it.

■ The soft spot on top of your baby's head (the fontanelle) may be tight or bulging.

■ The baby may seem irritable and may dislike being handled.

■ The body may be floppy or else stiff with jerky movements.

Remember, a fever may not be present in the early stages.

Older children may have slightly different symptoms.

■ A constant generalised headache.

■ A high temperature, although hands and feet may be cold.

■ Vomiting.

■ Drowsiness.

■ Confusion.

■ Sensitivity to bright lights, daylight or even the TV.

■ Neck stiffness – moving their chin to their chest will be very painful at the back of the neck.

■ A rash of red or purple spots or bruises which does not fade when you press a glass tumbler or finger against it. The rash may not be present in the early stages.

■ Joint or muscle pain.

■ Rapid breathing.

■ Stomach pain, sometimes with diarrhoea.

Symptoms can appear in any order and not everyone gets all the symptoms.

**Causes** There are different types of meningitis which can be caused by either bacteria or viruses.

**Prevention** Vaccinations against haemophilus influenzae (Hib) and meningococcus C, two types of meningitis, are now part of the childhood vaccination programme. Both are safe and extremely effective. Some forms of meningitis do not, as yet, have a vaccination so the disease can still happen. It pays to keep an open mind.

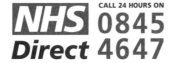

**NHS Direct** CALL 24 HOURS ON 0845 4647

**More information** The National Meningitis Trust provides free information to sufferers of meningitis and their relatives. Their 24-hour support line is 0345 538118. The Meningitis Research Foundation also has a free 24-hour helpline which provides help and information to the public and health professionals. You can phone them on 080 8800 3344.

**Note** People who have been in contact with someone who has had meningitis should contact a close relative of the patient to find out any instructions (from the hospital or the Director of Public Health) that they may have been given. Otherwise your doctor will be able to give you appropriate advice. Only people who have been in very close contact with the infected person are given antibiotics and vaccination.

## Menopause

*Menopause is a natural part of life and not a sign of illness. As the number of eggs released from the ovaries reduces, your periods become irregular, shorter and eventually stop altogether. There is no 'normal' age for this to happen and it can range from 40 years to 58 years. The average age for the menopause is around 51. A quarter of women will experience no difference except the lack of periods, half will report mild changes and a further quarter will experience marked changes in the way they feel, along with physical differences.*

### Symptoms

Not all women will experience these physical symptoms and their severity will also vary. Even how long the symptoms last will range from a few months to a few years. Symptoms include:

- hot flushes;
- vaginal dryness;
- pain when having sex (mainly due to dryness);
- sweating;
- headaches;
- an irregular heartbeat; and
- joint pain.

As with physical symptoms, the non-physical changes also vary greatly between women, but include:

- irritability;
- depression;
- tiredness; and
- poor concentration.

These can all lead to a lack of confidence, worries over the future, poor sleep patterns and strains on relationships.

**Causes** The changes in hormonal states, particularly the drop in oestrogen levels, are the biggest factors. However, not all problems experienced around the menopause are due to a lack of oestrogen. Many problems can relate to the general effects of ageing, anxiety, or changes in people's lives.

**Menopause continued**

**Prevention** Talk to your doctor about the advantages and disadvantages of hormone replacement therapy (HRT). Many of the early claims for HRT have not been supported by evidence over time. On the other hand, the scares over HRT have also been found to be exaggerated in many cases. Leaving aside any possible improvement in the symptoms of menopause, HRT does help prevent osteoporosis. On the downside, it may slightly increase your risk of breast or uterine cancers. Do not rush into any treatment. Ask first about all the risks, with or without HRT, and the risks of any alternatives, so you know all the facts before making a decision.

**Complications** The most important medical complication is osteoporosis (a thinning of the bones). You should report any vaginal bleeding, no matter how small, to your doctor if it happens after your periods have stopped for good.

### Self-care

■ Regular exercise is valuable in maintaining muscle tone and beating depression. Aim for any activity which leaves you slightly breathless, such as walking or cycling. Even 15 minutes a day will make a huge difference.

■ Vaginal lubricants will improve your lovemaking, but remember to use water-based lubricants if you or your partner are using condoms.

■ Continue to use contraception for two years after your last period if it ended while you were under 50 years old. Otherwise, use contraception for one year.

■ You may find certain drinks trigger your hot flushes. Thankfully, night sweats get better, but it can help to change your nightwear.

## Migraine

*Migraine is common and runs in the family.*

### Symptoms

■ Visual patterns, such as chequerboards or spots, are often a warning of an attack. Migraine can make you feel weak, sick and not able to concentrate.

**Causes** The exact cause is still not known, although there is some connection with the blood vessels of the skull. Certain foods appear to trigger migraine. Red wine, particularly Chianti, blue cheeses and chocolate are all culprits. Stress, the weather and even hormonal changes have been known to increase suffering.

**Prevention** Avoid triggers such as red wine or blue cheese.

**Complications** The greatest danger from headaches is missing something more serious than the common causes. Irritability increases along with a shorter fuse. There is a greater risk of having an accident, as well as a risk of overdosing on paracetamol.

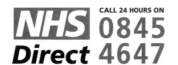

CALL 24 HOURS ON
**NHS Direct** 0845 4647

### Self-care

■ Light can hurt the eyes and lying in a darkened room helps for some people, although some doctors believe it is better to just get on with 'normal' life if possible. The attack can last from a few minutes to a few days. You can get treatments from your doctor which may reduce or even prevent a full-blown migraine attack. Anti-inflammatory drugs (for example, ibuprofen) can help ease the pain and are generally better than simple painkillers. (Do not take ibuprofen if you are pregnant.)

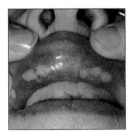

# Mouth ulcers

*Ulcers in the mouth are very common. Most are harmless and will clear up on their own. Unfortunately, some ulcers may be more serious and may need the attention of your dentist or doctor. There are different types of ulcer; the most common is the aphthous ulcer which is seen most often in teenagers or in women just before their period. Teeth with jagged edges or badly-fitting dentures will also cause ulcers, particularly on the gums and cheeks.*

### Symptoms

■ Aphthous ulcers are small, white and usually less than pinhead-sized with a red border and, despite being particularly painful, will disappear within a week or so. They usually appear on the inside of the lower lip or inside the cheeks. Drinking something hot or acidic, such as orange juice, usually makes their presence known. Ulcers from teeth or dentures are usually larger and get bigger rather than disappear. Any ulcer that fails to get better should be seen by a dentist or doctor.

**Causes**  Aphthous ulcers can appear at any time but are more common during times of stress or when you are run-down. Constant rubbing from a tooth, filling, dental plate or dentures will also cause an ulcer. Tongue and mouth cancer is extremely rare in young people.

**Prevention**  Except for checking your dentures and looking after them correctly, there is no real way of preventing mouth ulcers. For people who often get mouth ulcers, a lack of vitamins may cause them. Regular dental checkups will make sure that any persistent ulcer is sorted out.

**Complications**  Ulcers from teeth or dentures can become infected, making eating even more painful.

### Self-care

■ If you wear dentures, make sure they fit properly. Ulcers may get better by themselves, but if you find the pain is too much, salt-water rinses, mouthwashes or rinses containing chlorhexidine can reduce pain and help your ulcers to heal more quickly. There is no evidence that other antibacterial mouthwashes work. There is some evidence that corticosteroid paste rubbed onto the ulcers can reduce pain and help quicker healing. You can get these treatments from the pharmacy. Gels that numb the pain can ease the discomfort but have no effect on healing time. If the ulcer has not gone after three weeks, see your dentist or doctor.

**Action**  See your pharmacist or dentist or call **NHS Direct**.

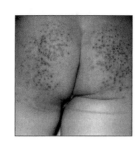

# Nappy rash

*Rashes in the nappy area are common but can be reduced or avoided completely.*

### Symptoms

■ The rash is usually red, not raised, and confined to the nappy area.

**Causes**  It is caused by the irritating effect of urine and bowel motions. If they are cleaned away quickly enough, or the baby is allowed to have the nappy off for a while, the rash will not appear.

**Prevention**  As far as is possible, change each nappy after it has become dirty. Remember that urine can be every bit as irritating as faeces (poo). Avoid disposable wipes containing alcohol or moisturising chemicals. Instead, use plenty of warm water. As much as possible leave the nappy off, particularly plastic pants. Dry, cool skin rarely forms a nappy rash. You should wash reusable nappies according to the manufacturer's instructions. Avoid caustic household detergents.

**Complications**  An angry red rash which does not respond to treatment or spreads beyond the nappy area may be a fungal infection (Candida). You need an antifungal cream and may need an oral antifungal agent as it often starts in the mouth. Ask your pharmacist or doctor.

### Self-care

■ Quickly treat any rash that appears with ointment from your pharmacist.

■ Avoid talcum powder generally as it can cake badly and cause even more irritation.

# Peptic ulcers

*Gastric ulcers affect the lining of the stomach and are more common in people over 40. Using high doses of steroids over a long time, for example, for asthma or rheumatic conditions, can cause a gastric ulcer. Even relatively small doses of anti-inflammatory drugs, such as ibuprofen or aspirin, can lead to an ulcer in the stomach in people who are prone to ulcers. Duodenal ulcers, which are found lower down in the abdomen, are more common in men. They heal more easily than the gastric type and usually develop just at the beginning of the duodenum.*

### Symptoms

■ The symptoms of peptic ulcers tend to overlap but there is a fairly general pattern.

*Gastric ulcers*

■ Constant pain or cramps can happen, which are particularly bad after eating (eating tends to settle pain in a duodenal ulcer).

■ Indigestion remedies (antacids) often settle the pain but it usually comes back.

■ Belching (burping) is common and embarrassing.

■ Vomiting can happen.

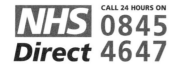

### Duodenal ulcers

■ Most people know they have developed a duodenal ulcer at around 2am when they wake with a pain like a red-hot poker just above the belly button.

■ Drinking milk can help but hot spicy foods make it much worse. Eating small amounts of food often relieves the pain.

**Causes** Ulcers may be caused by a bacterium called Helicobacter that lives in the stomach. Your doctor can check for this. Stress, smoking and alcohol abuse may also be causes.

**Prevention** Avoid smoking, too much alcohol and 'rich' foods. Milk and indigestion remedies (antacids) do help.

### Complications

Call your doctor if there is:

– blood or brown soil-like blood in your vomit;

– black tar-like blood or fresh red blood in your bowel motions;

– severe pain just below the ribcage;

– dizziness when standing up; or

– a strong thirst.

### Self-care

■ Most peptic ulcers will respond well to treatment with modern drugs which reduce the amount of stomach acid. You can also help ease the pain by using indigestion remedies or antacids.

**Note** If the pain has just started but is lasting more than a week, despite medicines from your pharmacist, call your doctor.

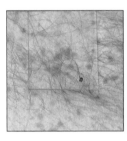

## Purpura

*Serious problems are rare. These irregularly-shaped, dark-red spots could follow an allergic reaction to infection or some disorder of the blood.*

### Symptoms

■ The spots are not usually irritating, range from around pinhead size to a couple of centimetres (around one inch), tend to come and go and will not fade when pressed with a glass tumbler or a finger.

**Causes** Children between two and 10 are most likely to be affected. There are a number of causes but anything that affects the ability of the blood to clot can cause this rash.

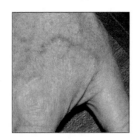

## Ringworm (tinea)

*Ringworm (tinea) can affect many parts of the body, particularly the groin and scalp.*

### Symptoms

- It is most noticeable on bare skin when it is known as ringworm due to its characteristic appearance as a circular patch of red, itchy skin, which gradually increases in size.
- There may also be red, itchy areas around the base of hair shafts.
- With scratching, these areas can bleed and become crusted with blood.

**Causes**  It is not a worm, simply a fungus (tinea).

**Prevention**  Keep the area well ventilated and dry. Use a separate face cloth and towel – ringworm is infectious.

**Complications**  Bacterial infection from scratching is common.

### Self-care

- Keep the area well ventilated and dry.
- Use a cream or special shampoo, as recommended by your pharmacist.

## Scabies

*Although intensely itchy, scabies is rarely a serious condition.*

### Symptoms

- Red lines which follow the burrows of the mite as it travels in the skin soon blend together. It is usually worse at night when the mite is most active.

**Causes**  Scabies is caused by a mite which burrows just under the skin, often between the fingers, on wrists, elbows and the genital areas, causing a red rash. It can only come from contact with infected people.

**Prevention**  It is very difficult to prevent.

**Complications**  Bacterial infection from too much scratching can make the situation worse.

### Self-care

- Use lotions or creams which you can get from your pharmacist. All of the body will need to be covered with the ointment for 24 hours and all clothing and bedding should be washed thoroughly.

**NHS Direct**  CALL 24 HOURS ON **0845 4647**

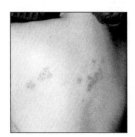

## Shingles

*One step up from cold sores, shingles is caused by a closely related virus. It is particularly nasty if the immune system is not working properly, during illness or while on treatment for cancer. It is rare to develop shingles more than once.*

### Symptoms

- A tingling itchy feeling happens before a painful rash appears.
- It is only found on one side of the body.
- It can develop over the next few hours or days into a painful set of blisters.
- It usually follows a narrow strip of skin. Common sites include the chest wall, face and upper legs.
- A general flu-like illness often comes with the rash, which may last after the rash has gone.

**Causes** If you have never had chickenpox, you are very unlikely to develop shingles which is caused by the same virus.

**Prevention** It is difficult to prevent. Most people will develop the infection without realising where it came from.

**Complications** Although sometimes very painful, shingles is rarely serious. People who are suffering from any condition or medicine which lowers their resistance to infection can be quite ill. If it spreads onto the tip of the nose, it may affect the eye and you should see your doctor immediately.

### Self-care

- Once the tingling sensation begins, it is wise to start using an antiviral medicine or acyclovir (for example, Zovirax).
- Simple painkillers, such as aspirin and paracetamol, help.
- Keep the rash area uncovered as much as possible.
- Try not to scratch the rash. Use calamine lotion to ease the itchiness.
- Pain which follows the disappearance of the rash can be reduced by cooling the area with a bag of ice.

### See your doctor, especially if:

- the outbreak of blisters happens near your eye or at the tip of your nose;
- you also have a sore red eye;
- the sores have not healed after 10 days;
- you also have a high temperature; or
- you suffer from some other serious illness.

**More information** Although it is possible to treat the infection with acyclovir (for example, Zovirax), it is important to start treatment as soon as possible when the itchiness first starts. Once the rash is well developed, acyclovir is unlikely to help.

## Smoking and lung cancer

*Lung cancer was rare until tobacco hit the scene.*

– *This is the most common type of cancer in men, with over 100 new cases for every 100,000 men diagnosed each year in the UK. 31% of all deaths from any cancer are from lung cancer. 30,000 men develop it each year, compared with 14,000 women, but women are catching up. More women than men smoke, most of them young women.*

– *The peak age for lung cancer is between 65 and 75. It is relatively rare below the age of 40.*

– *Only 8% of people survive lung cancer.*

– *Tobacco smoking in its various forms is the single biggest cause.*

– *The more cigarettes smoked and the younger the age at which smoking started, the greater the risk.*

– *Cigar and pipe smokers have a lower chance of developing lung cancer, but their risk is still higher than for non-smokers.*

– *Inhalation of tobacco smoke by non-smokers – known as passive smoking – has also been shown to be a risk factor for lung cancer.*

### Symptoms

You should go to your GP if you:

■ have a cough that won't go away;

■ have coughed up blood; or

■ are increasingly short of breath.

**Causes**  Smoking causes lung cancer. Full stop.

**Prevention**  Giving up smoking or, better still, not starting in the first place, makes sense. Around 100 people die every day from lung cancer. The good news is that stopping smoking works. A study has shown that stopping before middle age avoids more than 90% of the health risks of smoking.

### Self-care

■ Research shows that using nicotine replacement therapy products will double your chance of successfully quitting. Nicotine patches, gum, inhalers and so on can now be prescribed by your GP, or bought over the counter in pharmacies and in some supermarkets. The non-nicotine drug, Zyban, can also help smokers to quit. Zyban is only available on prescription and is not suitable for some people, so it is essential you discuss it with your doctor before it is prescribed.

■ There is plenty of free help and support available on the NHS when you want to stop smoking, and remember that people who use professional support are more likely to be successful in their attempts to quit. Your local NHS Stop Smoking Service provides a range of free services to help you stop smoking, including one-to-one and group support. Call the NHS Smoking Helpline on 0800 169 0 169 to find the service nearest to you.

■ If you can't do it for yourself, do it for your partner or kids.

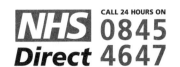

Quit plan:

- Choose a stress-free day to stop. Tell friends and relatives – they will support you.
- Get someone to give up with you. You will reinforce each other's willpower.
- Clear the house and your pockets of any packets of cigarettes or tobacco, papers or matches.
- Take it one day at a time.
- Map out your progress on a chart or calendar. Keep the money you have saved in a separate container.
- Chew on a carrot. It helps you do something with your mouth and hands.
- At first, avoid events where you may be tempted to smoke.
- Keep busy. Being physically active will help reduce cravings.

## More information

NHS Smoking Helpline
0800 169 0 169
Lines are open seven days a week from 7am to 11pm.
Specialist advisors are available from 10am to 11pm.

NHS Pregnancy Smoking Helpline
0800 169 9 169
Lines are open seven days a week from 12 noon to 9pm.

NHS Asian Tobacco Helpline
Lines are open from 1pm to 9pm every Tuesday.
0800 169 0 881 – (Urdu)
0800 169 0 882 – (Punjabi)
0800 169 0 883 – (Hindi)
0800 169 0 884 – (Gujerati)
0800 169 0 885 – (Bengali)
Website: www.givingupsmoking.co.uk

## Note

- Within eight hours, the oxygen level in your blood increases to a normal level. Chances of a heart attack start to fall.
- Within 24 hours, carbon monoxide leaves the body. The lungs start to clear out mucus and debris.
- Within 48 hours, nicotine is no longer found in the body. Your sense of smell will become stronger, as will your sense of taste.
- Within three days, spasm of lung tissue reduces, making breathing easier. Lung capacity increases.
- Within three months, your circulation has improved, walking becomes easier and even your liver begins to improve. Most of the detoxification of the nasties absorbed from smoke takes place in the liver.
- Within ten years, your risk of lung cancer has dropped dramatically, some doctors say by up to 50%.

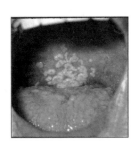

## Oral thrush in adults

*Candida albicans, a yeast fungus, will grow in the mouth if the body's natural resistance lowers or if there is a change in the natural balance between the microbes which normally live in the mouth.*

### Symptoms

■ Sore, creamy yellow patches on the inner cheeks and throat, which leave a raw area when rubbed (for instance, when cleaning teeth).

**Causes** Some medicines, such as steroids, or repeated courses of antibiotics can allow thrush to form in the mouth. It can also result from a lowered immune resistance from some medical conditions such as diabetes or, more rarely, AIDS.

**Prevention** Good oral hygiene, using antibiotics correctly and not having too many antibacterial lozenges all reduce your risk of oral thrush.

**Complications** Oral thrush can cause denture problems such as raw areas under the plates. As it is rare in adults, you should get medical advice to check for any underlying condition.

### Self-care

■ You may need a course of antifungal drops to clear the fungus.

**Note** If the thrush keeps returning, you should get medical advice.

**Action** Ring **NHS Direct** or ask your pharmacist.

## Oral thrush in children

*Candida albicans, a yeast fungus, is more common in young children and babies, where there is often no apparent reason for it to grow, although it is encouraged by repeated courses of antibiotics.*

### Symptoms

■ Sore, creamy yellow patches on the inner cheeks and throat, which leave a raw area when rubbed.

**Causes** Although a lowered resistance to infection caused by some medicines or medical conditions is a factor, oral thrush is so common in babies that it is very rarely a sign of anything serious.

**Prevention** Breast-feeding may give some protection from infections generally.

**Complications** Babies can have difficulty feeding and may cry, particularly if drinking fruit juice.

### Self-care

■ A course of antifungal drops may be needed to clear the infection.

**Note** If the thrush keeps returning, you should get medical advice.

**Action** Call **NHS Direct** or ask your pharmacist.

**NHS Direct**

CALL 24 HOURS ON
**0845 4647**

# *Vaginal thrush*

*Candida albicans is a fungus which should not normally be present in large numbers in the vagina. For various reasons it can grow rapidly and cause thrush.*

## Symptoms

- A creamy, thick white vaginal discharge.
- Itchiness and irritation.
- Pain or burning after passing water.

## Causes

- A prolonged course of antibiotics.
- The oral contraceptive pill. Hormonal changes before a period.
- Steroid treatment.
- Diabetes.
- Immune system problems.
- Sexual intercourse with an infected man.

**Prevention**  After being on the toilet, wipe from front to back. Change underwear often, particularly after exercise. Choose cotton rather than nylon pants. Avoid harsh soaps as they kill the good bacteria which prevent thrush.

**Complications**  Thankfully, there are few serious complications of thrush. It can, however, make life very miserable. Sex is painful, as is passing water.

## Self-care

- Eat live yoghurt and apply it to the vaginal area. It will replace the missing lactobacillus which prevents thrush.
- Ask your pharmacist for antifungal preparations.
- Your partner may need treatment as well.

## Note

See your doctor if:

- thrush does not disappear after self-care or keeps coming back for no apparent reason;
- the discharge changes in smell or appearance; or
- there is any abdominal pain.

# Contraception

## Planned parenthood

As well as deciding whether to have a family, men and women are also deciding on the size of any family they want to have. People should become parents by choice, and the decision must be a joint agreement. Planned parenthood is clearly better for all concerned – you, your partner, your children – than unplanned parenthood.

## Which contraception is for me?

There are a number of different methods of contraception, each of which has its advantages and disadvantages. All forms of contraception work by preventing the fertilisation of a woman's egg by a man's sperm. This can be achieved in various ways.

- One approach is the barrier method, which physically prevents sperm from swimming into the uterus and fertilising the woman's egg.
- Another approach is the hormonal method, which alters a woman's hormonal cycle to prevent fertilisation.

Other types of contraception include the following.

- The intrauterine device (IUCD), generally used by 'older women' (older women in the reproductive sense are quite young in the general sense). The IUCD is not recommended for young women who have not had children.
- Natural methods, which are often not effective enough.
- Sterilisation, which is a permanent surgical procedure and can be very difficult to reverse if you ever decide to have children in the future.

Obviously, these types of contraception are not really suited to younger people.

All the hormonal methods of contraception are available from a doctor or family planning specialist. Some barrier methods, such as the IUCD, are available only from a doctor, but others, such as the condom and spermicides, are widely available in pharmacies (chemists), toilets, supermarkets and family planning clinics. Another great advantage of barrier methods of contraception is that, if used properly every time, they also provide protection against sexually-transmitted infections (STIs) such as chlamydia and HIV.

- Everyone is entitled to free and confidential advice even if they are under 16.
- Contraception is free even if you are under 16.

## Barrier methods of contraception

The barrier methods of contraception include the male condom, the female condom, the cap, the diaphragm and spermicides in the form of foam.

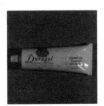 *Contraceptive gel*

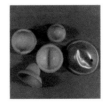 *Cervical caps (various sizes) (left) and the diaphragm (right)*

**NHS** CALL 24 HOURS ON
**Direct** 0845 4647

### The male condom

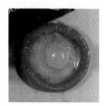

Society is increasingly accepting the condom as one of the normal requirements of modern life. This has led to wider availability, and condoms are now readily available in supermarkets, from garages and through slot machines, as well as in pharmacies. Colours and flavours make interesting options. Some condoms are lubricated with spermicide, which increases their effectiveness as a contraceptive and provides a degree of protection from STIs (sexually-transmitted infections). Even in a stable relationship, the protection provided by condoms can be valuable, as thrush (Candida) is a common infection of the genital tract for both men and women, particularly after prolonged courses of antibiotics, and can be sexually transmitted. If sealed correctly, the modern condom will remain usable for a long time (look for the Kitemark of the British Standards Institute). Once the seal is broken, the condom should be used quite soon, as the rubber will be ruined when it is exposed to the air and the lubricant will dry, making it difficult to put on.

**Using condoms**  Putting a condom on in the correct way is important. Air should be pushed out from the end of the condom as it can cause it to burst or slip off when the penis shrinks in size after ejaculation. Sharp fingernails are a hazard, and only the soft fingertips should be used to unroll the condom onto the penis.

### Spontaneity

Perhaps the single biggest stated reason for not using condoms is the widely-held belief that they make unplanned sex difficult. Foreplay is an important part of enjoyable sexual activity and partners can involve condoms in this way. Fears that they reduce the sensitivity of sexual experience have not been supported by experiment. The problem is the psychological inhibition some men have over their use.

### The female condom

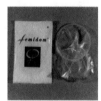

The condom for women is relatively new, but regular users report favourably and many men prefer it to the male condom. It is much larger in diameter than the male condom and has two flexible rings, one at each end. The smaller ring fits inside the vagina while the outer, much larger ring stays on the outside of the vagina. After ejaculation this outer ring should be twisted and gently withdrawn to prevent sperm escaping.

### The female contraceptive pill (oral contraceptive)

Mixed hormonal contraceptive pills mimic pregnancy, which reduce the release of hormones that stimulate the final development and release of ova (eggs) from the ovary. This partly explains why some women suffer the milder symptoms of pregnancy while they are using the pills.

The progestogen-only pill discourages sperm from getting anywhere near the womb by maintaining the natural plug in the neck of the cervix, which will not allow the passage of sperm while the levels of progesterone are high. This pill has many of the advantages of the mixed pill without the 'pregnancy'. However, you have to take it regularly at the same time each day.

# Contraception continued

While the contraceptive pill is convenient and relatively efficient, there are definite health risks associated with its use – especially if a woman smokes, is overweight, or has a history of either heart disease, high blood pressure, liver disease or high cholesterol levels. Women over the age of 35 can often take the pill safely, but doctors will consider whether other risk factors are present in deciding whether to prescribe this form of contraception.

### Intrauterine contraceptive device (IUCD)

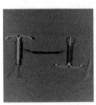 This small plastic device, inserted by GPs or doctors at family planning clinics, causes a mild inflammation within the womb which makes the lining of the womb unsuitable for the fertilised egg to implant itself. It can be left in the uterus (womb) for up to five years, although the newer versions that release a measured amount of progesterone (see the oral contraceptive pill) need to be checked every year. Most doctors recommend an IUCD to be used only after the first pregnancy, as there is a small risk of infection, which can lead to infertility. The device is removed very easily by a doctor and has no effect on sensation during sex.

### Hormone implants for women

Based on the same principle as the progestogen-only pill, it is possible to insert, under a local anaesthetic, very small containers of the hormone just beneath the skin. The hormone discharges itself at a set rate, providing total contraception for around five years.

### The male pill

Male contraception is still being developed. A male oral contraceptive pill has yet to be passed as safe for human use in the UK, although there have been successful trials in China and encouraging results in animal experimentation.

### Vasectomy

As a form of contraception, vasectomy has maintained its position as a popular, almost 100%-sure way of preventing unwanted pregnancies. It is, along with the condom, one of the very few ways in which a man really does have control over conception. For most men, its single biggest attraction is that it doesn't interfere with the actual enjoyment of sex, while providing as near absolute contraception as possible.

**Risks**  There have been reports of an increase in the possibility of testicular cancer in men with a vasectomy, but the risks, if present, are extremely small. There is a similar risk of impotence, which has also received attention in the press. All these reports must be considered in perspective. Your decision will depend on your age, how many children you already have and the effect any further children may have on your family. Doctors are obviously not keen to perform a vasectomy on men who do not have any children.

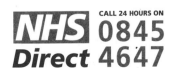

**NHS** CALL 24 HOURS ON **0845**
**Direct** **4647**

**The operation** The operation is relatively simple. Basically, the vas deferens, which carries sperm from the testes to the penis, is cut and tied off or clipped at both cut ends. This effectively prevents any sperm from reaching the penis. A small cut is made through the skin of the scrotum, under either a local or a general anaesthetic. Once identified, each vas is cut, a small piece is removed and the cut ends are tied off. Each segment that has been cut away is sent off to the laboratory to make sure that the correct tubes have been treated and that there is no sign of any serious medical condition that needs attention. Using a couple of stitches or staples, the wound is closed. It takes no more than about 15 minutes and is extremely safe. Testes do not swell from sperm building up in them, nor shrink away from lack of use.

**100%?** Nature can tell when a normal body function has been interfered with. There are a number of cases, thankfully very few, where a successful operation has been confirmed with a definite removal of the vas tissue and yet a few years later the man concerned has fathered a child. It appears that the body is capable of overcoming surgical intervention by creating fresh canals for the sperm to travel to the penis. It has to be said that the risk is extremely small, but it explains why the form you sign agreeing to the operation points out that it will not guarantee 100% success.

## Emergency contraception

If you have had sex without using contraception, or think your contraception might have failed, you can use 'emergency' contraception. You should not use this as a planned method of contraception. 'Emergency' contraception, either in the form of the so-called 'morning after' pill – which must be used within 72 hours of unprotected sex – or by inserting a coil within five days, should only ever be used in an emergency. If you act quickly, 'emergency' contraception can usually prevent pregnancy.

## Natural methods

Theoretically, it is only possible for a woman to conceive within seven days of ovulation or 24 hours afterwards. Using various tests it is possible to estimate the time of ovulation.

You can do this by keeping an eye on and recording the following signs on each day of your menstrual cycle.

■ Your body temperature first thing in the morning (before any exercise, food, drink or even smoking). By using a thermometer and a chart, it is possible to detect the sudden rise in temperature of around 0.5 degree Celsius that takes place at ovulation. Obviously, this can be confused by increases in temperature from a cold or flu. The 'safe' phase begins on the morning of the third day of increased temperature.

■ Cervical mucus – Testing your cervical mucus helps to define the beginning and end of your fertile period. During the fertile time, the cervical mucus becomes clearer, wetter, stretchy and slippery like raw egg white.

■ The length of your menstrual cycle – This helps to define the time you are fertile. Record your last six menstrual cycles. From these records, find your shortest cycle and take off 20 days to find your first fertile day.

Compared with the other methods described, the 'natural' method is not very safe and you need to have self-control and good record-keeping. This method is most effective when discussed and explained to you by your doctor, a practice nurse or a specialist in family planning.

# Sexually-transmitted infections

Sexually-transmitted infections (STIs) can affect you at any age, whether you're straight or gay, in a long-term relationship or with a casual partner. Symptoms don't always show up immediately, so you could have been infected recently or a long time ago. It is important to make sure that you always practise safer sex by using a condom. If you haven't practised safer sex, you can have a confidential checkup and treatment, if needed, at a genito-urinary medicine (GUM) or STI clinic. Call **NHS Direct** for details of your nearest clinic.

## Chlamydia

Non-specific urethritis, which simply means an inflammation or infection of the urethra, is a term which includes infection by chlamydia. Men and women suffering from this infection may complain of an intense burning sensation when passing water. There may also be a white discharge. It actually causes few problems for men other than this discomfort but can be disastrous if it is passed on to women. This condition is often free of symptoms in women. It is not only the single biggest cause of infection of the Fallopian tubes (pelvic inflammatory disease), leading to infertility and ectopic pregnancy (a potentially lethal condition where the baby attaches to the wall of the Fallopian tube instead of the wall of the womb), but can cause blindness and pneumonia in a child born to an infected woman. Condoms provide almost total protection.

**Treatment**  Chlamydia is treatable with antibiotics.

## Hepatitis B

Although hepatitis B is one of the more deadly sexually-transmitted diseases, there is now a protective vaccine to prevent it. Even so, the number of infected people is rising steadily and stands at roughly 700 people each year. It can cause as little as a flu-like illness or as much as total destruction of the liver. Typically, it will cause different degrees of jaundice (yellowing of the skin and the whites of the eyes). This is caused by the build-up of a pigment which is normally broken down by the liver.

Most people will not need immunisation but, depending on your lifestyle, it may be wise to speak to your GP. It is transmitted in the same way as HIV, that is, by bodily fluids. It only needs a tiny fraction of a drop of blood to transmit the disease. For this reason it can be caught from sharing a toothbrush or kissing when there is bleeding from the gums. Worse still, the virus can survive a week or more in the dried state and so can be picked up from, for instance, a razor. There is no way of knowing if the person you are having sex with has the infection. The incubation period, that is, how long it takes before the illness appears, is six months from the time of infection. Some people can 'carry' the virus and not know.

## Genital herpes

This is the third most common STI. Roughly 50% of people who have had one attack never have another. Unfortunately, it is impossible to completely get rid of the virus. Herpes Simplex Virus (HSV) comes in two forms, HSV I and HSV II. Both infect the same places and are likely to infect parts of the body where two types of skin meet together. Both forms can infect the corners of the mouth, the outer parts of the genital areas and even the anus. Both cause crusted blisters and then ulcers that weep a thin, watery substance. This substance is highly infectious, since it contains the virus that causes the condition. Herpes comes in attacks which can last for months and then disappear for years, or even never return. You are definitely infectious while you still have the sores. Even when sores are not present, it might be possible to pass on the infection. Other illnesses and stress can bring on these attacks. For some people, the condition will pass unnoticed, with only tiny ulcers on the penis to show its presence.

**Treatment** Anti-viral drugs can be applied directly to the affected skin or taken orally. They are most effective if they are used before the sores break out. This is signalled by a tingling, itchy, painful sensation in the affected area. They are only effective during the first attack in some people and have not been shown to have any effect on later attacks. Condoms with a spermicide appear to offer greater protection than those without. You need to arrange your sex life around the condition if you are having an attack, as this means you are highly infectious. Otherwise, using condoms gives maximum protection for your partner.

## Genital warts

Papilloma viruses, which cause warts, can affect any part of the skin. The virus can be transmitted by physical contact, including sex. Like the warts commonly seen on people's hands, they can vary in size from tiny skin tags to large fungating masses like cauliflowers. One in eight people going to GUM clinics has genital warts. Around 100,000 people are treated for these warts each year in the UK, many more may simply put up with them, and many people do not even know they have them. They may be a factor in causing cervical cancer in women and rectal cancer in gay men.

**Treatment** There are drugs which can be applied directly to warts which will cause them to disappear. Liquid nitrogen is now used less often as it can leave a painful 'burn' in such sensitive areas. Genital warts usually cause little discomfort, although they are often itchy and may bleed with scratching. Use a condom to prevent catching them in the first place.

## Syphilis

Syphilis is a potentially serious condition. It is caused by a spirochete, a microscopic parasite, which is highly infectious. Most people are unaware of the infection but if it is not treated, it can develop over a number of years into a condition which can affect the brain. Women show few signs of the infection in the early stages, except for small ulcers around the vagina, so it can go unnoticed by the woman or by her partner during intercourse. The parasite cannot pass through a condom, so this will give almost 100% protection.

**Treatment** Penicillin that is given as a single large dose can be given by injection and should cure the condition if it is caught in the early stages.

# Sexually-transmitted infections continued

### Trichomoniasis

Causing a yellow or green discharge from the penis or vagina, this microscopic parasite lives in the urinary tract and usually causes pain when passing water but can sometimes have no symptoms. When it has no effect on the male partner but the female partner complains of a smelly green discharge from the vagina, tests may show its presence in the man.

**Treatment**  The parasite is sensitive to the antibiotic metronidazole.

### Gonorrhoea

Caused by bacteria, this disease is commonly misdiagnosed as it can often give only a few symptoms. It is commonly known as 'the clap' from the French word *clapoir,* meaning sexual sore. Gonorrhoea is not rare. It can cause a yellow or white discharge from the penis or vagina, along with pain on passing water. When it infects the anus, there can be a similar discharge. Most of the symptoms of infection will start within five days of infection and include a vague ache of the joints and muscles. Although these can disappear after a further 10 or so days, the person is still infectious. It can make it harder for women to conceive if it is not treated.

**Treatment**  Antibiotics are usually effective. Condoms provide almost 100% protection from infection.

### Thrush

See **Oral thrush in adults** on page 114 and **Vaginal thrush** on page 115.

### Your choice for treatment

You can go to either your own doctor or the local genito-urinary medical clinic (GUM), which is located at one of the major hospitals in your area. Confidentiality is all-important at these clinics. You will need to be honest with the doctor who asks you questions, as it can be impossible to work out what is wrong without the correct information. You can give a false name or no name at all if you feel more comfortable, although there is no chance of anyone finding out you have been to the clinic (not even your GP) or finding out about the results of any tests.

You may need to have certain tests to get an accurate diagnosis, although it may be fairly obvious on your first visit, and the treatment may start immediately without you having to go back. It is worth remembering that the doctors and nurses who staff these clinics are professionals who see you as simply a person who, like any other patient, needs treatment.

**NHS Direct**  CALL 24 HOURS ON **0845 4647**

# Weight loss

**(Over 4.5kg (10lbs) in 10 weeks without dieting or trying to lose weight.)**

Losing weight, or at least trying to lose weight, is very popular at the moment. This is perfectly reasonable if you are overweight, but there should be a good reason why you are seeing the pounds drop off. A significant loss of weight for no good reason is not normal. Increasing exercise will reduce your weight as long as you are not eating more than usual. Cutting down on alcohol if you have been drinking too much will also trim your waistline. But if you are losing weight and cannot pin down exactly why, you should be aware of some medical conditions which include weight loss in their list of signs and symptoms.

Do you, for instance, have an increased thirst, pass water more often and feel generally tired? Some hormone deficiencies, such as diabetes, can cause weight loss with these symptoms. This condition tends to run in families so if a close relative suffered from diabetes, it will increase your risk. A simple test can be performed by your practice nurse.

Feeling restless, sweating a lot, feeling weak and having difficulty sleeping may be the signs of a hyperactive thyroid gland, which is producing too much thyroxine. This will cause weight loss by increasing your basic metabolic rate. Again, a simple blood test can check this for you.

Some rare infections, like tuberculosis, and even rarer disorders of the immune system, such as AIDS, can also cause weight loss. It is possible for your doctor to check for these conditions in a number of ways, including blood tests and X-rays.

Persistent diarrhoea with unusually pale stools may mean you are not absorbing your food properly. This may be due to an inflammation of the digestive system. Any marked changes in your bowel habit (how often you pass a motion) or any blood or tar-like substances in your stool can be caused by inflammation or a tumour. You may not always get abdominal pain, although if you are in pain, there is even more reason to get it checked sooner rather than later.

www.nhsdirect.nhs.uk

# Healthy living

Life is to be enjoyed and could be much more pleasant if we were all healthier and lived longer to enjoy it. Simple things can make a big difference and don't mean a complete change in the way you live. Here are some tips on how to stay healthy and live longer, without worrying about it.

## Eating for pleasure and health

An increasing number of people are becoming overweight. We know this can increase your risk of heart disease so cutting down on fatty food, especially animal fats, makes sense. Simply grilling food rather than frying it will significantly reduce the amount of fat you are eating.

Some foods are known to reduce your risk of many illnesses and possibly even cancer, yet are cheap and taste good. Fruit supplies vitamins and fibre and can replace sweets for children, especially as a 'treat' or reward. Aim for around five servings of fruit or vegetables each day. (One serving is roughly one piece of fruit, one dessert bowl of salad, one glass of fruit juice or two tablespoonfuls of vegetables.)

Try gradually cutting down on salt with your food. You'll be surprised how little you need after getting used to less. It will protect you from high blood pressure.
Fish, especially the oily varieties such as mackerel or sardines, are loaded with special oils which actually protect your heart. Bread, especially wholemeal types, potatoes and pasta are all great forms of carbohydrate which provide energy and should be the main part of the meal. Enjoy your food and go for as wide a variety as possible.

## In a puff of smoke

The more we look at smoking and health, the more we know that cigarettes are the single greatest killer in our society. Over 300 people die every day from smoking-related diseases. Smoking 25 cigarettes a day increases your risk from lung cancer by a staggering 25 times. It also doubles your chances of heart disease.

- Get someone to give up with you and name the day to start.

- One day at a time is the best plan, but reward yourself each day by, for example, putting the money you normally spend on cigarettes in a jar.

- Tell people in the pub or at work that you are trying to stop. These days they will understand and support you.

- Get rid of all the tobacco stuff in the house, like ashtrays, lighters and matches.

- See your pharmacist about nicotine replacement which will help ease the cravings.

For more information on giving up smoking go to ***Smoking and lung cancer*** on pages 112 and 113.

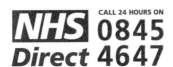

**NHS Direct** CALL 24 HOURS ON 0845 4647

## Are you active?

Most people think they are more active than they actually are. Even a small amount of exercise or physical activity will help protect you from heart disease, which is still the greatest cause of death. Aim for at least 15 minutes every day of activity which leaves you slightly breathless. You don't need to buy expensive machines or even go to gyms or leisure centres.

- Take the stairs instead of the lift.
- Get off the bus one stop early and walk quickly.
- Play with the children. Being a 'horse' for them gets your heart pumping.
- Climb briskly up the house stairs.
- If possible, cycle rather than take the bus or use the car. Most towns are making special tracks for cyclists.

If you are out of doors in the sun, make sure your head is covered and you have a high-factor sunscreen (SPF15 or higher).

## Sexual health

The UK has the highest rate of teenage pregnancies in Europe. At the same time sexually-transmitted disease is on the increase. Using simple protective contraception like male or female condoms would help protect against unwanted pregnancy and sexually-transmitted infections such as HIV (AIDS).

- Condoms are on sale in supermarkets and chemists, and you can get them free from your family planning clinic.
- Don't take anyone's word for it – insist on using a condom if you are not in a well-established relationship. Gay men should use the extra-strong variety.
- Emergency contraception ('morning after' pill) will reduce the chances of pregnancy but it won't protect you from infections. Condoms will.
- Emergency contraception must be taken within three days (72 hours) of unprotected sex. Call **NHS Direct**, your family planning clinic, your local genito-urinary clinic or your GP to find out where to get it.

## Alcohol

Relatively recently we have found out that moderate drinking for men and women over 40 can actually help prevent heart disease. The problem is that the message gets confused and there is a temptation to drink too much without realising that this protection is very soon lost as the amount of alcohol consumed rises. To make matters worse, women are more at risk from the harmful effects of alcohol than are men and it's not just a matter of average body size. Aim for no more than three to four units of alcohol a day if you are a man and slightly less, two to three units, if you are a woman. Alcohol abuse is on the increase and children are drinking heavily at a much earlier age, setting the pattern for later life.

One unit of alcohol is roughly the same as: ■ an English measure (25ml) of spirit (Scotland and Northern Ireland use larger measures); ■ half a pint of normal-strength beer; ■ one measure of sherry (50ml); ■ one small glass of wine (100ml).

Some beers are very strong and we all pour out more generous measures at home. Cans and bottles bought in supermarkets are labelled with the number of units of alcohol they contain.

If you would like more information or advice about alcohol, you can call Drinkline free and confidentially on 0800 917 8282. The helpline is open Tuesday to Thursday 9am to 11pm and 9am to 9pm Friday to Monday.

www.nhsdirect.nhs.uk

# What are your risks?

Some dangers to health and life are very serious but the risk of actually suffering from them may be very small. These risks can be difficult to work out, especially as the press tends to highlight particular risks to health, making them appear more likely to happen than they do.

It can also be very confusing trying to compare risks. For example, **the risk of being killed by lightning in the UK is 1 in 10 million people a year**. This doesn't mean very much to most of us. So try thinking about it in this way.

At a risk of 1 in 10 million you would need a line of people 10,000 kilometres (6,000 miles) long to contain the single person who would be killed by lightning. It would take four months of non-stop walking to reach the end.

On the other hand, **the risk of death from smoking 10 cigarettes a day is just over 1 in 100 people a year**. The line of people would now only be 100 metres (110 yards) long and it would only take you two minutes to reach the end.

### Reducing risks

Some of the risks to health cannot be easily avoided. Many are so small it makes little point even trying to do so. There are some risks, however, which are not only quite high but also partly or totally avoidable. Cigarette smoking is a good example. Although there is still a risk from inhaling other people's smoke (passive smoking), the chances of your health being affected are far, far greater by actually smoking yourself. Another example is the number of deaths from flu which is also small (1 in 10,000 people a year) but is higher in elderly or ill people. These 'at risk' groups can lower their risk by simply having a flu vaccination (the 'flu jab').

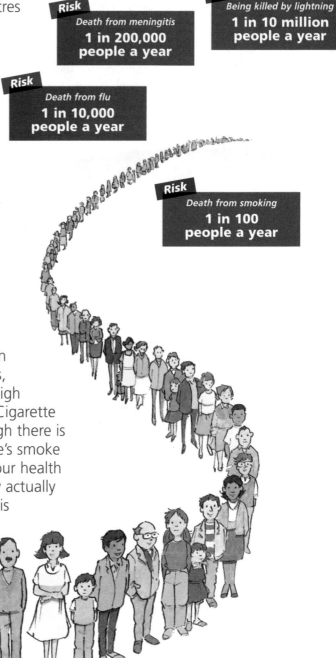

Risk
Death from meningitis
**1 in 200,000 people a year**

Risk
Being killed by lightning
**1 in 10 million people a year**

Risk
Death from flu
**1 in 10,000 people a year**

Risk
Death from smoking
**1 in 100 people a year**

**NHS Direct**

CALL 24 HOURS ON

**0845 4647**

126

# Medicine chest

Minor illnesses or accidents can happen at any time so it's worth being prepared. It makes sense to keep some first aid and simple remedies in a safe place to treat minor complaints and accidents.

- Paracetamol and aspirin (children under 16 and people with asthma should not take aspirin)

- Paracetamol (for example, Calpol) or ibuprofen syrups (or both) for children

- Mild laxatives

- Anti-diarrhoeal medicines

- Rehydration mixture

- Indigestion remedy (for example, antacids)

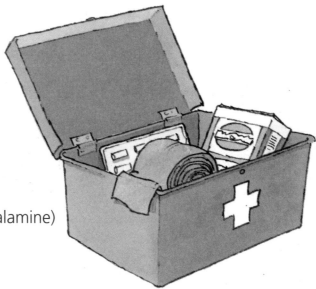

- Travel sickness tablets

- Sunscreen – SPF15 or higher

- Sunburn treatment (for example, calamine)

- Tweezers and sharp scissors

- A thermometer

- A selection of plasters, non-absorbent cotton wool, elastic bandages and dressings

## Remember

- Keep the medicine chest in a secure, locked place, out of reach of small children.

- Always read the instructions and use the suggested dose.

- Watch expiry dates – don't keep or use medicines past their sell-by date.

- Take all unwanted and out-of-date medicines back to the pharmacy. This is to stop medicines getting into the water supply and the wrong people getting hold of medicines someone else has thrown away.

# What is an emergency?

When it comes to your health or the health of someone in your family, it is often very obvious if the person is seriously ill and needs immediate emergency care.

An emergency is 'a critical or life-threatening situation'. That's all very well, but it still doesn't really help you decide what a 'critical situation' is. Here are some examples.

- Unconsciousness
- Heavy blood loss
- Suspected broken bones
- A deep wound such as a stab wound
- A suspected heart attack
- Difficulty in breathing

There are a few things that you should remember in any emergency. These will help you to deal with the situation quickly and efficiently.

- Stay calm.
- Do everything you can to help the person, but don't put yourself in danger.
- Don't give the person anything to eat, drink or smoke.
- Don't stick anything in their mouth.

## How can you help them?

The way to help a person very often depends on what is wrong with them. Sometimes, the quickest way to help is to take the person to the nearest accident and emergency department. This will vary from area to area as it does depend on how close your local hospital is. However, even in an area where your hospital is fairly close, you should call an ambulance and not move the patient if:

- you think they may have hurt their back or neck, or may have any other injury that may be made worse by moving them;
- the person is in shock and needs your constant attention; or
- the person has severe chest pain or difficulty breathing.

## The recovery position

If the patient is unconscious, there is a safe position to put them in which allows them to breathe easily and stops them choking on any vomit. Once you have checked that they are breathing normally, lie them on one side, with a cushion at their back, bring their knee forward, and point their head downward to allow any vomit to escape without them swallowing it or breathing it in. Remember, when you are moving the patient onto their side, make sure their neck and back do not move.

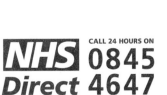

**NHS** CALL 24 HOURS ON
**Direct** 0845 4647

## Some myths about Accident and Emergency services

- **Accident and Emergency is an alternative to your GP.** *False*
  It is not appropriate to go to Accident and Emergency as an alternative to your GP.

- **Calling 999 for an ambulance gets you to the top of the Accident and Emergency queue.** *False*
  Patients are seen based on medical need, not who gets to the hospital first.

- **All injuries need X-rays.** *False*
  The doctor or nurse will be able to assess, on examining you, whether an X-ray is appropriate or not. In many cases X-rays are not needed.

- **Accident and Emergency doctors are more expert at dealing with medical problems than your GP.** *False*
  Your GP is an expert in general medicine. Accident and Emergency doctors are specialists in accidents and emergencies.

- **Taking pain relief before being seen by a doctor will 'mask' the symptoms of the injury.** *False*
  One of the first things that is often done by doctors is to give you a simple painkiller like paracetamol. It is quite safe to take these before you get medical advice. Taking pain relief to treat minor injuries is the best way to make you feel better quickly and is an effective treatment. Always follow the instructions on the packet.

## Some myths about GP services

- **Your doctor has to visit you at home.** *False*
  If a home visit is appropriate, the doctor or nurse will arrange it. Doctors decide whether or not to visit a patient at home, based on your medical need. Only patients who cannot reasonably come into the surgery are visited at home.

- **You will be seen more quickly if you ask for a home visit.** *False*
  During surgery hours, most doctors visit patients later in the day. It may be quicker for you to go into the surgery during normal surgery hours and out of hours. If you do the travelling, it means that the doctor can see more patients rather than spending time travelling themselves and delaying your consultation.

- **All infections need antibiotics.** *False*
  Antibiotics have no effect on most infections (such as colds, flu and most sore throats) because viruses cause them. Taking too many antibiotics can lead to new bacteria developing which cannot be killed by antibiotics, which is dangerous for individual people and for the whole population. Doctors recommend that you visit your pharmacist for over-the-counter remedies for minor complaints.

www.nhsdirect.nhs.uk

# Index